THE AUSTRALIAN MASSAGE

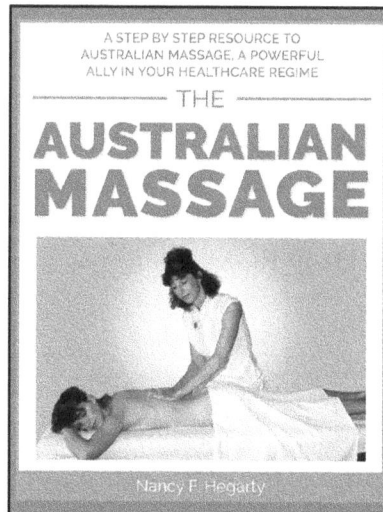

A STEP BY STEP RESOURCE TO
AUSTRALIAN MASSAGE, A POWERFUL
ALLY IN YOUR HEALTHCARE REGIME

THE

AUSTRALIAN MASSAGE

Nancy F. Hegarty

Nancy F. Hegarty

First Edition: 1993

Second Edition: 2015

National Library of Australia Cataloguing-in-Publication entry: (paperback)

Creator: Hegarty, Nancy F., author.
Title: The Australian massage / Nancy F. Hegarty
ISBN: 9780992403461 (paperback)
ISBN: 9780992403409 (ebook)
ISBN: 9780992403485 (CD-ROM / DVD-ROM)
Subjects: Massage--Technique.
        Massage--Australia.
        Massage therapy.
Other Creators/Contributors: Hegarty, Peter J.E.
Dewey Number: 615.822

Publisher
Paradise Waters Pty Ltd
P.O. Box 1856, Innisfail,
Queensland, Australia 4860

For enquiries, write to: rights and permissions, refer publisher.

Dedication

I dedicate this offering to all who have taught me what I know, and to Divine Intelligence for guiding me to write this book for you who love to learn in a skilful manner, making this an even better world to live in and enjoy every day, knowing that love and peace are what our bodies thrive on.

Disclaimer

The author of this book does not dispense medical advice nor prescribe the use of any technique as a form of treatment for medical problems without the advice of a health professional, either directly or indirectly. This book is not intended as a substitute for medical recommendations of healthcare providers. The intent is to offer information to help the reader co-operate with health professionals in a mutual request for optimum well-being.

Because any material can be misused, the author and publisher are not responsible for any adverse effects or consequences resulting from the use of any of the procedures suggested in this book. The author disclaims any liability in connection with the use of this information.

The publisher and author are not responsible for any goods and/or services offered or referred to in this book and expressly disclaim all liability in connection with the fulfilment of orders for any such goods and/or services and for any damage, loss or expense to the person or property arising out of or relating to them.

The publisher and author cannot accept responsibility for any mishap resulting from the use of any remedy described in this book. The ideas, procedures and suggestions contained in this book are not intended to replace the services of a trained health professional.

Nancy F. Hegarty

CDs

Daily Relaxation Meditation

Pain Management & Preparation for Healing (Meditation)

Meditation for Mustering Intensive Energy

An Introduction to a Healthy Life (positive affirmations to music with beats)

e-Books

The Australian Massage

Simple Foods to Heal Your Body

The Australian Advanced and Metaphysical Massage

BOOKS

The Australian Massage

Simple Foods to Heal Your Body

The Australian Advanced and Metaphysical Massage

DVD

The Australian Massage Therapy

Acknowledgements

I acknowledge with joy and pleasure:

My father, Stan Newitt (1910 – 1984) and mother Chyril Newitt (1929 – 2013) for resolving my bodily cramps with instinctive massage in 1969, and then after my father's passing 'to the other side' a small inheritance from his estate contributed to therapeutic massage studies and my first natural health centre

Queensland College of Massage Therapy for initially sharing an abundance of knowledge with me, Principal Allan Sirett, QINS, BSSM, ARMTO (Bach), J.P. (1987)

My many clients, students and teachers in the field

Oswald Henry (deceased), World Reporter and Editor of medical magazines for his encouragement and photographs of Diploma and Certificates

Sharon Salvestrin, my daughter for her effervescent support as Teacher's Aid in Bundaberg during the early stages of my college of therapeutic massage, 1990

TAFE College at Craigie and Wanneroo Recreation Centres in Perth, Western Australia for providing support and encouragement to share with others that which I strongly believe

Steve Hegarty, my husband who enjoyed modelling for photographs in The Australian Massage book, for providing unending support and most importantly his clarity and strength

Foreword

Regardless of the description of a good body massage (pampering, rejuvenating, therapeutic) or the reasons we seek it (luxurious retreat, stress relief, pain management), when performed holistically and as instructed throughout this book, without a doubt, it is a powerful ally in our healthcare regime.

Massage as a healing tool in many cultures has been around for many thousands of years. Touching is a natural human reaction to pain and stress, conveying compassion and support. Healers throughout time have instinctively and independently developed a wide range of therapeutic techniques using touch. Research indicates that up to 90% of disease is stress-related and massage is a perfect elixir for good health, providing an integration of body and mind. Instructed by one of the best teachers in the natural health field, Nancy shows the many incredible benefits that are doubly powerful, providing emotional and spiritual balance and true relaxation with inner peace.

The Australian Massage is a non-invasive, humanistic and drug-free method based on the fundamental principle of the body's natural ability to heal itself. Each movement has a scientific process, all adding up to a world of good. To the everyday person, the professional massage practitioner and everyone in between who is looking to improve their well-being skills I personally recommend this wonderful method. While enhancing a positive self-image, moreover, it makes you feel good!

Sharon L. Salvestrin
Director of Romantic Retreats
www.romanticretreats.com.au

Introduction

After reading through The Australian Massage you will not only understand how to perform a professional therapeutic massage, you will also learn what to look for in an honourable massage room, and also discover if an establishment that conducts massage is reputable.

Having travelled extensively and received therapeutic massages in many countries, I notice even today there is a distinct necessity for professionalism still to be learned, applied and respected. Numerous places provide a high level of cleanliness and care and there are always those that have room for a little or lots of improvement. As for the massage movements, practitioners who I have found using an obvious knowledge of anatomy and physiology during the massage treatment are trained to a very high standard, Certificate IV level. There are also those who have read anatomy and physiology however choose not to apply this knowledge in their movements.

There are far too many that continually rub, rub, rub and continue to rub so much more on an area of the body, whether that be muscle, joint or/and bone, or where there is noticeable stiffness until the receiver is left with bruising or intense discomfort, not only on the couch (or for up to 48 hours later as you may be told) but for many days or weeks later. If you can relate to that, find another. There are many who also discover a sore spot and repeatedly rub or dig into it. In most cases it is felt when the sciatic nerve in the lower torso region or a nerve in another area of the body is deeply pressed. This is not what a good massage treatment is about. It is all about the end result - balance - of the body, mind and spirit. In my next book, The Australian Advanced and Metaphysical Massage there is a great deal of information that will assist in understanding what can be expected during a remedial, lymphatic or kinesiology treatment.

Some establishments leave the receiver with the belief that massage therapy provides the best natural healing on earth and the receiver feels totally synchronised with the body. That is how it is meant to feel. There are others that will leave the receiver with a degree of uncertainty because the receiver has experienced a non-professional massage treatment.

Consider this. You are having a massage treatment and your partner is waiting for you in the lounge of the establishment. A book is chosen from the selection on a table close by for example, The Art of Sensual Massage. Now imagine that this is the wife having a massage and the husband is with the book. He simply cannot put it down as his eyes are glued to the pictures of a naked man and a naked woman on a bed, not just any bed but one that is luxuriously presented. Something had to be well-dressed for the scene. A man is intimately stroking the woman in the pictures. The husband continues turning the pages. He looks up every so often to see if anyone is looking at him perusing this book's contents. What thoughts could be now going through the husband's mind? His wife is out of sight in the hands of he doesn't know who? What is he expected to think when a book such as this is in the waiting room? How do you think I felt when seeing a book of similarity in a chiropractor's business where a registered massage therapist had his shingle up too? This practitioner was professional and well respected. Reading material with such explicitness has its private place and that is not in a practitioner's waiting room. It does nothing to maintain the professional wellbeing of those therapists who are genuine. That very incident planted firmly in my mind that this book had to be re-written and set free into the world.

After many years of giving my jolly best, most other massages now leave me feeling somewhat lacking at the end of a treatment due to an exceptionally high level of expectation. There are a few that shone above all others and there are many good practitioners. There are some places throughout this world, even up to 5 star rated hotels that employ qualified therapists who wear uniforms, are scrupulously clean and the practitioner is totally dedicated, and there are those that have left me concerned about their methods, cleanliness and/or personal care of the receiver. Maybe the efforts that are coming from within can always be improved by listening to one of my positively affirmed meditations. What about the unsuspecting person who experiences for the very first time a non-professional massage treatment?

There are places that teach their 'therapists' in the massage room with no formal qualifications necessary. It is not always the case that high rating hotels only hire Diploma level practitioners either which came as a complete surprise. Then there are places that you never know just what you are going to receive until you enter the premises. If something doesn't feel quite right to you, ask questions and follow your gut feeling, leaving if necessary.

If you feel unsure, ask to see the practitioner's credentials. If one is not readily available and you accept a treatment then please do not expect that all practitioners thereafter will also give the same quality of service.

There are also some registered, professional practitioners who need to be scrutinised. You can do some pre-treatment qualifying first. Does the room feel comfortable to be in? Is it clean? What does it smell of? Does the practitioner wear a uniform? Are qualifications on display or readily available? Does the practitioner belong to a registered body of professionals in the natural health industry? Are you offered a large towel, covering garment/s or disposable underwear to wear while waiting for the practitioner and during the treatment? Do you have complete privacy to change?

Are the practitioner's fingernails short and clean? How does the practitioner's breath smell to you – any lingering alcohol, smoke or simply outright putrid? If so, really, how dedicated to the body is that practitioner? Is the practitioner polite? These are a few basic pre-requisites that may guide you to a good quality professional practitioner and of course to receiving a professional massage treatment. In Australia, if you have private health insurance extra cover, upon the receipt of a fully qualified and registered practitioner's paid invoice you may be entitled to receive a rebate. Ask before the treatment if it is claimable through your specific health fund.

You are never in doubt after you have experienced a professional massage by a good practitioner. Your body feels balanced. Your 'sore' bits will no doubt feel improved in some way now that you feel totally in sync with life. Your body begins to appreciate how you take care of it. Your whole life's outlook changes for the better. You feel happier to be alive. Your happy thoughts create your healthy body and you are so grateful.

If seeking to become a professional massage practitioner in Australia you will need to be trained by a Certificate IV level provider.

To further your education in advanced massage therapy The Australian Advanced and Metaphysical Massage as an instructional manual is available.

The Australian Massage is recommended for readers 18 years of age or over.

The Australian Massage is here for you to experience and enjoy. You will find it is easy to follow and learn when applied with patience and a wholesome, healing attitude. What you provide from your heart to your giving hands is the vital key to your successful end result. Massage therapy only works when this is the driving force behind caring professional movements.

Contents

Preface

The easiest way to begin learning The Australian Massage is by reading through the chapters so you have a general idea of what to expect. Next look closely at each photograph. Practice hand positions and movements before the actual applications. Write down the steps to enhance your memory of the sequence then begin with the most important of all, a willing partner in need of pain relief.

A good Anatomy and Physiology reference book beside you will assist in locating specific muscles, bones, tendons and ligaments. The Advanced Australian and Metaphysical Massage contains more detailed diagrams that can be of assistance.

The application of The Australian Back Massage on a monthly basis may increase the opportunities of improved well-being and therefore greater productivity in your chosen profession. The cost of these services whether funded by the recipient, employer, a private health fund or government could very well lead to an overall reduction in the cost of health care over time. Natural health practitioners who apply these techniques as instructed certainly believe so.

Prior to learning the method, Part One through to Part Six discusses what you can do prior to commencing, what massage oils are best to use, emotional responses, overall benefits, when to and when not to apply The Australian Massage movements, privacy, basic movements and also shows the general location of major bones and muscles of the body.

Because of the intricacy in movements Part Seven (Chapter One through to Chapter Five) explicitly explains and shows the method in close-up photographic detail of:

- The Australian Back Massage
- The Back of the Legs
- Arms, Wrists, Hands and Shoulders
- The Front of the Legs
- Ankles and Feet
- Neck and Head

Chapter Six gives you Quick Tips for ready reference when applying this method and in Chapter Seven essential oils are briefly discussed, including herbs and their applications with references to further studies.

Remember, if you are having any difficulties following these instructions The Australian Massage video that was originally filmed in 1990 and produced at Burnett Studios in Bundaberg shows everything you will need to know about this specialised method. This method is also available on DVD.

PART ONE

PRIOR TO COMMENCEMENT

THE ROOM
MUSIC
AROMA

THE COUCH

COMFORT
MEASUREMENTS
DRESSING THE COUCH
MAKING THE SHEET

CLOTHING AND
PERSONAL GROOMING

UNIFORM
SHOES
HYGIENE

PRIOR TO COMMENCEMENT

Etiquette

Restrain pets or animals from the entry point to the massage room and make sure they cannot demand your attention by scratching on doors.

Visitors or people in close proximity must be quiet and respectful when the receiver is having a massage treatment.

Ensure all mobile phones and other electronic communication devices are switched off or out of hearing distance from the massage room. If one must be close by, switch off any ring tone or mute potential sounds and never answer it during a massage.

The Room

Ensure that the temperature in the treatment room is around 24º - 25º Celcius or is comfortable for you to work in. If it is at 22º - 23º Celcius make certain you have enough large towels on standby to use as blankets. Towels are easy to wash. Blankets are difficult to maintain. Linen must be clean and fresh for every person. If the room is too warm for you, cool to suit your working conditions ensuring the receiver's warmth is taken care of by covering with an extra towel or two. Ask the receiver to inform you if feeling too cool or too hot so you can attend to their comfort.

About half way through the massage, the recipient's body temperature will have begun to lower so be aware of their comfort. The receiver may have forgotten what you said earlier. Ask her/him again to let you know if they feel too cool and if so add an extra layer of cover for warmth. On the other hand if too warm do your best to assist in maintaining the coolness appropriate for her/his comfort such as offering or applying a cool face washer to the face/forehead or hand towel to the hands /feet. Most times you will only need to apply a warm cloth when finished to remove any excess oil from feet and hands.

The room needs to have low lighting to avoid glare. If lights are bright, place an eye guard or soft, light cloth over the receiver's eyes when on their back. As you are practicing you will need plenty of light until you have learned the basic knowledge of anatomy and the method.

Music

Soothing soft background music aids in the relaxed atmosphere and also in the flow of your movements. Not only is gentle music soothing for the receiver, it also is good for you. Preferably a multiple CD, DVD or continuous play cassette player alleviates a mid-massage stop just to change the music or to turn the tape over, interrupting your continuous flow. There are very few tape players around these days. Most people have CD or DVD players or similar. The best music to use has no words. Music suitable for massage is available in "Recommendations", or you may prefer my CD, An Introduction To A Healthy Life, the most loving 286 life affirmations, the gift to creating miracles that is easy listening during a massage treatment (and also at home and play, or going to and from work). Both the receiver and you can experience the feelings of psychological freedom while preparing to continually create an enjoyable life. These gently plant new positive thoughts into your subconsciousness mind with beautiful music surrounding you.

Aroma

If you must fragrant the room by using a pottery or fireproof oil burner, place 1 mL of pure essential oil such as lavender for relaxing. Add 100mL of water to the oil heating dish. Place a lit candle underneath and let the delicate natural aroma fragrant the room. You may extinguish the flame just after you have applied the massage oil if the candle is within easy reach - without leaving the receiver of The Australian Massage. If you have chosen a basic plant oil such as cold-pressed coconut with added essential oil, this now allows the chosen aromatherapy oil blend to perform its task. If you have chosen basic non-aromatic oil, you may choose to leave the oil burner alight. Do not extinguish a candle in the presence of the receiver as the after- smell can be unpleasant. Unless you are working in the open air have an exhaust fan or window open that can readily remove the trail of smoke. Beeswax and soy candles are recommended.

The quickest and safest way to fragrant a room is with the use of a hot towel soaked in boiling water that has a few drops of essential oil added to it. This specialised technique is fully detailed in The Australian Advanced and Metaphysical Massage, "Hot Towel Application" where it is used on specific dis-eases.

The person giving the massage must advise the receiver what oil is going to be applied and needs to provide the option of an alternative. Ask if there are any known skin allergies. It is also advisable to give the receiver a whiff of the oil or blend you intend on applying. If the smell is pleasing to the olfactory system (sense of smell) this also provides a sense of well-being by infusing a sense of comfort.

THE COUCH

Comfort

A professional massage couch is very important for comfort both of yourself and the receiver. Ideally the couch top comes up to the joints between the wrists and fingers (where the metacarpals meet the phalanges) as you stand upright with arms loosely down by your sides. This correct height enables you to apply the method with the utmost of ease, ensuring a quality massage.

The most suitable couch is one with an opening for the receiver's head to rest in whilst lying face down. Check with the manufacturer on the shape of the hole before you order one. Where you live will help in choosing the best shape for the face hole. An oval or round shape may be more preferable. For added comfort use a small U-shaped pillow or roll a very soft hand towel and place it around the opening's upper and side edges.

Measurements

If you are making your own couch, the standard imperial measurements are 6 feet long x 2 feet wide or in metric is approximately 180cm x 60cm. In this case the oval hole's diameters are 5 inches across x 7 inches from top to bottom or 13cm x 18cm respectively. See where the hole is located on the couch diagram.

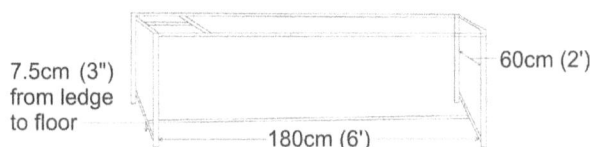

Couch Frame

Good quality soft vinyl is an ideal covering for your couch, padded with 2 inches or 5cm of very good quality foam. Cheap foam will not last and may crumble or crush after a short time of use. Good quality foam can last for twenty years. Add an extra ½ inch or 12mm foam strip between the top of the hole and the front edge of the couch for extra support. This will provide longer life for your couch top because this is where a lot of forehead movement and heat takes place which may flatten the foam.

Leverage bars approximately 3 inches or 7.5cm up from the floor and across each end are useful when applying the scalp movements, and neck and spine proprioceptive neuromuscular facilitation stretches (PNFs). It allows you to place one foot on the bar, providing stability when performing the PNF stretches (in The Australian Advanced and Metaphysical Massage). Use tubular iron and ensure to keep it protected with rustproof paint then finish with gloss enamel. Jazz it up with shiny silver, gold or whatever colour suits your décor. Best of all you could have a professional Feng Shui Consultation on your premises and use the best choice of Feng Shui prosperous or remedy colour as per the Flying Star Chart drawn and analysed by the Feng Shui Consultant.

To care for your couch use a cleaner that protects the covering as well as preserving the covering for the many years of use ahead. The last couch frame made for my centre was early 1991 by my husband, Steve. The couch top was covered with quality vinyl by a professional furniture upholsterer. It only retired from service in 2012 with no repairs to the top, only painting to change the frame colour to suit my day spa décor in 2006. The couch must be wiped with a gentle disinfectant cleaner after each use then immediately redressed in preparation for the next application of The Australian Massage.

Dressing the Couch

Cover the couch with a white sheet made to fit your couch. Have a large, neatly folded or rolled white towel ready for the receiver to cover with after disrobing to their undergarment. You could also place a disposable undergarment and hair net with the towel.

Making the Sheet

The sheet is quite simple to make if you have a domestic sewing machine and know the basics of sewing. Cut a white double or queen sized bed sheet in half, lengthways. Double hem around each raw side so there are no fraying threads exposed. Lay the sheet evenly over the couch. Take the outer corner, pulling tightly and ensure both sides are even. Pin the excess overhang into its final place, ready for sewing after the oval hole is cut.

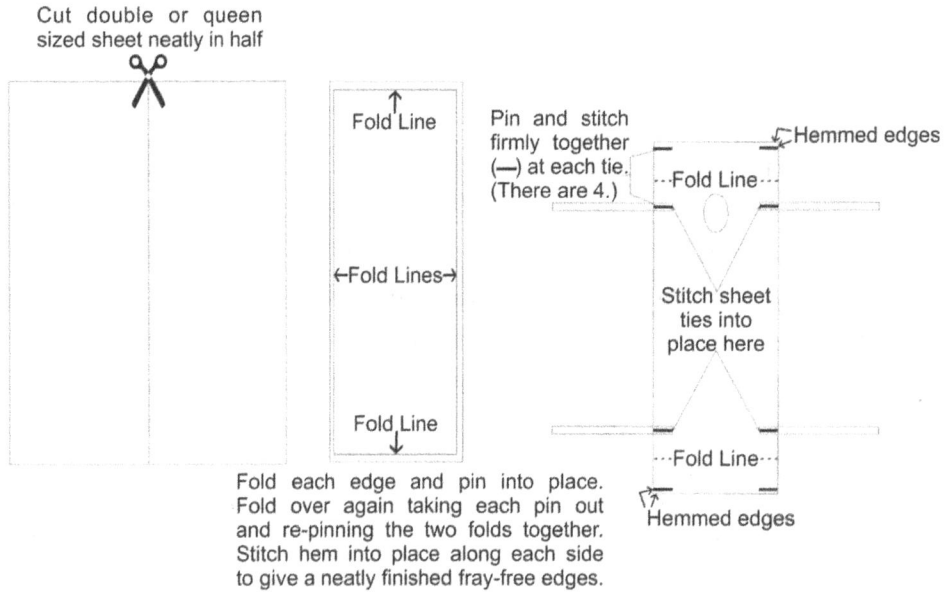

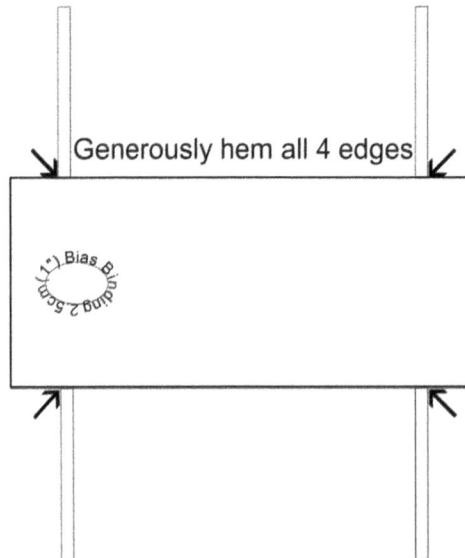

Cut double or queen sized sheet neatly in half

Fold Line

Pin and stitch firmly together (—) at each tie. (There are 4.)

Hemmed edges

···Fold Line···

←Fold Lines→

Stitch sheet ties into place here

Fold Line

···Fold Line···

Fold Line

Hemmed edges

Fold each edge and pin into place. Fold over again taking each pin out and re-pinning the two folds together. Stitch hem into place along each side to give a neatly finished fray-free edges.

Generously hem all 4 edges

Bias Binding 2.5cm (1")

Stitch a 60cm (2') strip onto the sheet
at the arrows
(for tying under the couch, keeping the sheet in place)

Using scissors cut a hole in the centre where the couch head hole is. Cut outwards making an oval shape leaving at least 5cm (2") spare of the actual couch hole's outline. Ensure you cut so that the opening is much smaller than the couch's head hole. If you cut to the same size as the opening the receiver's facial skin will touch the couch covering. This is not good for the longevity of the couch top because any facial perspiration may dry out the covering and also shorten the life of the stitching.

Using 2.5cm (1") bias binding as a facing, pin and sew this over the oval sheet edge covering all loose threads.

Holding the Sheet in Place

There is nothing more annoying when performing a therapeutic massage than to have a sheet that does not stay in its original position. Eliminate this by adding securing ties to the sheet. For extra holding stitch together lengthwise 4 x 2 60cm (2') lengths of bias binding. Pin each at the four sewing points (see arrows) of the four corners and sew altogether. With these strips tied into place under the couch at the top and the bottom you will always have a sheet that does not slide every way the receiver rolls and makes the massage a much smoother process. Whatever may have seemed like a minor problem was really a major discomfort. Resolving this is beneficial to both the recipient and the provider before commencing The Australian Massage.

CLOTHING AND PERSONAL GROOMING

Uniform

It is essential that you feel comfortable before you commence. Wear loose fitting clothing that allows for plenty of flexibility in your movements. Once you begin, your body will warm up so avoid overdressing. Offloading a pullover, cardigan or jacket after commencement is bothersome to both parties and can leave oil stains that will weaken your garment's fabric. In the event that you become a professional practitioner or are already qualified, wear a proper uniform that distinguishes your profession and ensure that it is laundered daily. Make sure the logo is visible. Never wear the same uniform you have worked in for two consecutive days. You may not be able to smell your body odour but others can, especially in such close proximity. In a very relaxed state near or at the end of a treatment the receiver's bodily senses are magnified and sense of smell is one of them.

If you are using certain vegetable oils you will soon discover that by placing your linen into a hot clothes dryer it will burn brown stains into your fabrics and render them useless for The Australian Massage. Beware of what oils you use. Look for least-staining oils. Although coconut oil is best taken internally or used in salads, and a little oil can be applied on the skin, it leaves clear staining and is virtually impossible to remove with normal cleaning practices. Repeated use of any vegetable oil can destroy the elasticity in a garment, some more so than others.

Many massage rooms smell of rancid oils, or towels are extremely heavy because the vegetable oils used are never removed completely from the linen. If those oils can be smelt on entering the room the practitioner needs to look at another way of laundering the linen to remove excess oil. I always recommend everything to be white thus enabling laundering to be carried out by professional cleaners in 60ºC hot water.

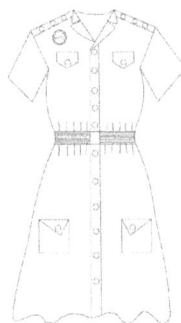

Add long sleeves (removable if possible) for winter warmth

Length is between knee and mid-calf with lots of width at bottom from gathering at waist. Conceal waist with band.

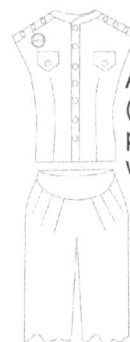

Culottes with large pleats for ease of movements Add longer legs for winter warmth

Designer Uniforms for Professional Female Practitioners

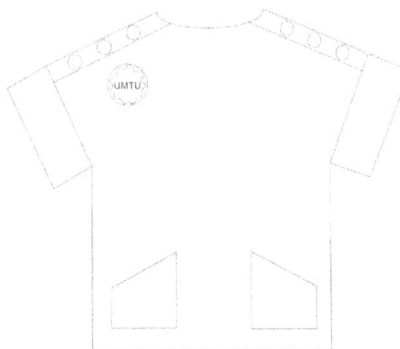

Lengthen or shorten sleeves and bottom hemline to suit

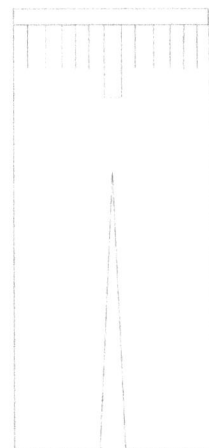

Lengthen or shorten to suit individual

Designer Uniforms for Professional Male Practitioners

Shoes

The Australian Massage is an excellent form of exercise so make the most of this by using as many of your bodily muscles as possible. It is very important that you maintain top health. The lighter your shoes are the better and make sure they are comfortable to wear. Shoes that hurt, squash and create discomfort to the feet produce diseased feet and in addition, silently forming facial wrinkles. Soft leather shoes with arch support are best. The internal material of the shoes is of a natural source (dependant on your location), e.g. cotton, wool, or leather and they are kept clean and well presented, always ready for each wear. Keep your shoes odour free. Wear short/long socks or some similar feet covering and change these once, twice or more times daily if you have a tendency to sweat.

Hygiene

Organic soap with Tea Tree oil has high antiseptic qualities and is one of the best hand cleansers. Your hands must be scrupulously clean and that means fingernails too. Keep these short and especially smooth with no rough edges. Check by running the ends of them over your own skin or if you have a piece of hosiery available this will certainly show pulls if there are any jagged edges on your nails. Now hold your palms facing you at eye level. If you can see any tip of your fingernail above the top of the finger or thumb it is too long for The Australian Massage and therefore this will sooner or later produce discomfort. Keep a nail file within easy reach and file each nail down to avoid unnecessary scratching on the receiver's skin. Ensure your teeth are cleaned and flossed at least twice daily and your breath is fresh. Avoid eating garlic as the pungency may be unbearable to the receiver. It can take up to two days for garlic breath to dissipate. The smell will not be noticed only if the receiver has also eaten garlic. I thoroughly recommend natural sugar free peppermint capsules be within easy reach and chew on one of these before a consultation. If using any type of gum safely dispose of before commencing any massage work. Take a look at yourself and see that you are neatly presented.

PART TWO

MASSAGE OILS
THERAPEUTIC MASSAGE OILS

THERAPEUTIC MASSAGE OILS

Quality

The Australian Massage oils are pre-mixed and placed where they are within easy reach. Once you begin The Australian Massage your hands do not leave the receiver's body so place the basic or blended oils close by on a surface that is easily wiped clean afterwards.

If you must use an essential oil always make sure it is pure and not the synthetic aromatic oils which may smell like the 'real thing'. They do not give the performance to the body. Many people believe that products smelling like flowers are made from natural ingredients derived directly from plants.

Understanding What a Fragrance is

Fragrance or parfum (a French word that means in our language, perfume) on a pretty bottle's label sounds lovely however please note: 95% of chemicals used are synthetic compounds derived from petroleum. "They include benzene derivatives, aldehydes and many other known toxics and sensitizers – capable of causing cancer, birth defects, central nervous system disorders and allergic reactions." (U.S. House of Representatives, 1986).

These synthetic chemicals go directly into the bloodstream when applied to the skin. Inhaling these chemical fumes go straight to the brain and some have a 'narcotic' effect. Most of the chemicals in fragrances consist of volitive organic compounds (VOCs) that are known to irritate the respiratory system. Inhaling fragrances can cause circulatory changes and electrical activity in the brain capable of also causing the inability to concentrate, dizziness, and fatigue (Fragrance Sensitivity, 2002).

According to the American Academy of Allergy, Asthma, Immunology (ACAAI) the vast majority of people with asthma have allergic reaction and a decline in lung function with synthetic fragrance exposure (Ziem, 2001).

An alarming discovery about the perfume industry is that it's not regulated at all, and any number of chemicals is able to be put into a fragrance without revealing what they are, and how these affect people. Try to avoid chemicals in the workspace.

Train your nose to recognise purity and quality from the very beginning. Begin with just one oil; e.g. lavender. You may find that five pure lavender oils each have a different aroma.

Do not apply essential oils directly onto the skin. They are strong, potent medicines when inexperienced in using them, with some oils being capable of burning not just the skin but also the breathing passages. Exacting quantities added to pharmaceutical carrier formulas produce the best results.

Pure essential oils are absorbed by the skin in one or two hours. Because of the certain qualities found in the oils, these can stimulate nail growth so keep a regular check on your nails. Remember to clean them before and after applying The Australian Massage.

If you are applying The Australian Massage on a regular basis using essential oil blends, for your own protection, wear close fitting surgical gloves. Your hands will absorb the oils too and over a long period of time, if you do enough applications of The Australian Massage (e.g. 5 to 30 per week) your own skin cells may begin to break down. It is the ailment of the receiver you are working on, not yours, so be aware for your own bodily protection.

If you are working indoors for most of the day see that your body soaks in some sunshine, at least five to ten minutes daily before 8.00am or after 5.00pm if in the tropics when permissible to help maintain healthy, glowing skin and strong bones. If in a moderate or colder climate these times are extended so will be much different. Where you live will determine safe times and how your body obtains vitamin D may be enhanced by your food intake.

Look For:

- Ingredients that do no harm to your skin and health
- A product that works and cares for your skin
- Plant and mineral based ingredients
- Environmentally friendly, including packaging
- Products for use on the skin with a pH of between 4.5 and 5.5 for adults and
- pH between 5.5 and 6 for babies and children

There are numerous companies now manufacturing much safer cleaning products than ever before however you need to access them either by phone/fax order or on-line such as Abode from www.cleanabode.com.au/ or www.shop.aces.edu.au. Other brands worth considering are Amaze Safe 'n' Clean, www.amazeproducts.com.au/, Sonett, www.sonett.com.au/, and Trinature, www.trinature.com.au/.

For organic personal care products you could try Aromababy, www.aromababy.com.au/ or Miessence, www.miessence.com, Aubrey Organics available in Queensland at www.innerglow. com.au. Also available are www.avalonorganics.com/, www.badgerbalm.com/, www.burtsbees. com.au/, www.cosmictree.ca/, www.drbronner.com.au/, www.earthtribe.com.au/, www. tomsofmaine.com/ and www.weleda.com/ to begin with.

You can have lots of fun exploring and discovering enjoyable ways to perform cleaning.

PART THREE

INDOOR AIR
GROW FRESH AIR
MOULD AND MOISTURE
DUST AND MITE CONTROL

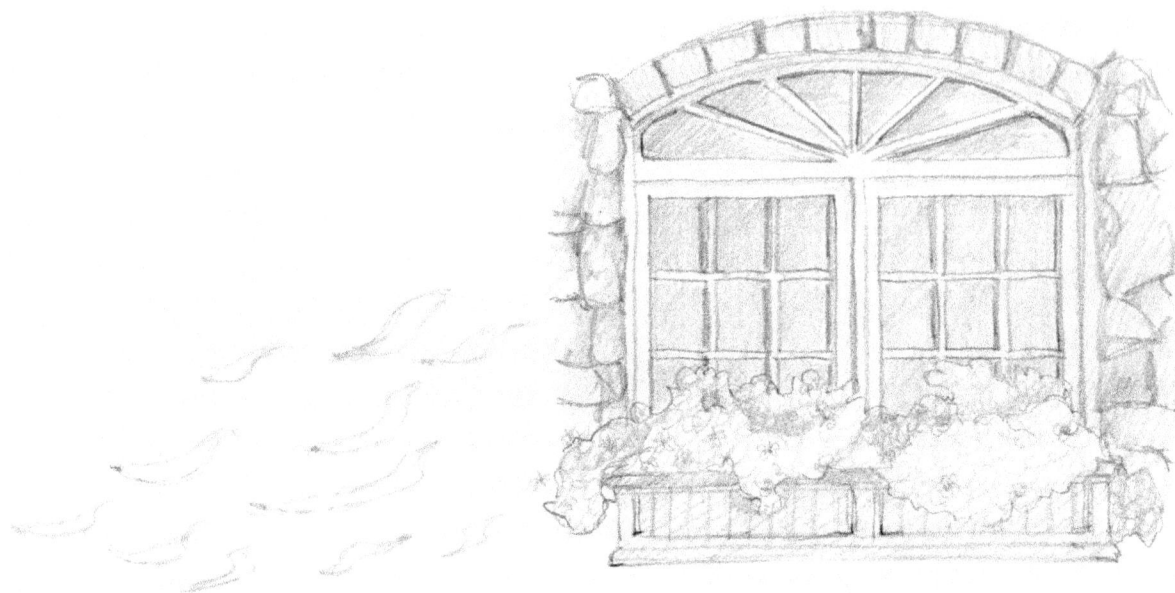

INDOOR AIR

Brominated flame retardants (BFRs) have routinely been added to consumer products for many decades to successfully reduce fire-related injury and property damage. Their polymers are used in computers, electronics and electrical equipment, televisions, textiles, foam furniture, insulating foam and other building materials. They are so pervasive that the dominant route of manifestation is household dust (Lorber, 2007). Apart from accumulating in the environment, there are serious concerns about their consequences on human health (Birnbaum and Staskal, 2004).

Formaldehyde is used in thousands of products as an adhesive, bonding agent and solvent and is classified as a volatile organic compound (VOC). VOCs are chemicals that become a gas at room temperature. Products made with formaldehyde will release the gas into the air and this is called off gassing. If high concentrations are off-gassed and breathed in, it could cause health problems (Minnesota Dept. of Health, 2011).

Formaldehyde is found in particle board, plywood, panelling, pressed-wood products, and urea formaldehyde (UF) foam insulation. UF resins are used as stiffeners, wrinkle resisters, water repellents, fire retardants and adhesive binders in floor coverings, carpet backings and permanent–press clothes.

Methods to lower the level of formaldehyde in a building:

- Allow new products to off-gas by leaving the product/s unsealed outside the premises such as an open shed for a few days.
- Increase ventilation by opening windows, turning on fans, or bringing in fresh air through a central ventilation system.
- Formaldehyde is water soluble and reacts to temperature changes. As the humidity and temperature go up so too does the amount of formaldehyde released from a product. The amount of formaldehyde off-gassing into the air is decreased by keeping the temperature and humidity low.

When present at levels above 0.1 parts per million parts of air, it has been known to cause a wide range of symptoms from burning sensations in the eyes, nose and throat, to nausea, coughing, and even skin rashes. Xylene and benzene from paints, lacquers, and mould inhibitors are among the other invisible gases that can cause a similar array of symptoms (National Cancer Institute, 2011).

Benzene is a commonly used solvent being present in many items including inks, oils, paints, plastics and rubber. It is also used in the manufacture of detergents, pharmaceuticals and dyes.

Grow Fresh Air

Indoor plants that absorb formaldehyde in the air include Nephrolepsis exaltata bostoniensis (Boston fern – very high and fast rate) and Dracaena marginata (the red-edged variety). Although Dracaena deremensis absorbs poisons and toxins in the air, NASA discovered Dracaena marginata to absorb best of these two. Dracaena deremensis (Janet Craig/ striped Dracaena) also removes a large amount of formaldehyde in household air, is especially effective in newly furnished rooms, and is one of the best at absorbing gaseous chemicals and any volatile organic compounds that are being released into the air from heated cleaners and fragrances (Shekut, Sue 2009).

More useful plants that may reduce air pollutants are Spathiphyllum (peace lily, also found very effective by NASA in purifying the air), Chamaedorea seifrizii (bamboo palm), Sansevieria trifasciata (mother-in-law's tongue) and Algaonema (Silver Queen or Silver King). Chlorophytum comosum (spider plant) may reduce mould.

Allow 2 to 3 healthy plants for every 30 square metres. Only water them when the top 2½ cm (1") becomes dry and give them a good soaking. By watering this way, it helps to leach the fertiliser salts out of the soil. Salt build-up is often responsible for browning leaf tips on many plants, especially spider plants and palms. Feed monthly with a high nitrogen plant food to keep them green and growing. Also bath their leaves' tops and under sides monthly either outside with the hose or in a shower (Rutherford, 2011).

English ivy (Hedera helix - best at removing benzene) and spider plant (Chlorophytum comosum – most effective at removing carbon monoxide) are inexpensive, ecologically sound, aesthetically pleasing ways to filter toxins from the building. Plants especially good at filtering certain pollutants are the areca palm (Chrysalidocarpus lutescens – most effective filter of xylene), crysanthemums, and dwarf date palms also help in removing formaldehyde (Yvonne, 2010).

Mould and Moisture

Moulds come in many colours, are a part of our natural environment and play a part in nature. Moulds are needed to break down dead plant and animal material and to recycle nutrients in the environment. Reproduction is by means of tiny spores that are invisible to the naked eye. These spores float through outdoor and indoor air. Moulds grow by digesting any organic matter such as leaves, wood, or paper and moisture. Without moisture mould cannot grow (California Department of Public Health, CDPH, 2011). Indoors mould growth needs to be avoided. Mould may begin growing indoors when mould spores land on wet surfaces. If mould spores are damp for any longer than two days mould begins to grow.

According to the United States Environmental Protection Agency (2012), moulds have the potential to cause health problems and can produce substances that can cause allergic reactions, irritants, and in some cases, potentially toxic substances. Some responses include sneezing, runny nose, red eyes, and skin rash and these are common. Allergic asthmatics can have an attack caused by moulds and according to CDPH, Indoor Air Quality Program, IAQP, (2011) moulds can also be the causation of new asthma.

Dust and Mite Control

Dust mites love warm and humid conditions. Even the cleanest home contains 1,000s of dust mites. Dust mites are microscopic eight legged arachnid insects that feed off dead skin cells (dust). The average human sheds about 10 grams of dead skin (or dander) per week, and domestic animals shed far more. The dust that the mites rely on is found in heavily concentrated amounts such as couches, recliners, children's toys, carpets, rugs, drapes, mattresses and linen, and in the air we breathe.

For many people dust mites are not harmful although they are the leading causes of allergies. It is not the mite itself or the dust that causes so many reactions such as allergic asthma, hay fever, eczema or conjunctivitis. It is the protein released in the dust mite droppings and decaying carcasses that is responsible for the allergenic effect in sensitive individuals (dust-mite.net, 2012).

There are several effective things that can be done to considerably reduce dust mites. It is virtually impossible to completely eliminate an inhabited building of dust. These are some ways to minimise dust and mites:

- Decrease humidity levels to less than 50% inside.
- Use a vacuum cleaner that has a High Efficiency Particulate Air (HEPA) filter. The best solution is to have a central vacuum system that vents to the outside of the building.
- Steam cleaning of carpets will kill existing dust mites. If you cannot replace carpeting heat-clean it at least once a year; and springtime is best. Replacing carpets with harder, impermeable surfaces is highly beneficial.
- Vacuum all fabric furniture including any drapes weekly with a HEPA filtered vacuum cleaner.
- Wash sheets, cushion and pillow covers with hot water for 15 minutes to kill existing mites at least fortnightly. Freeze small fabric items for several hours before washing them (Dust Mite Information Centre, 2004) e.g. toys, cushions or wash them in hot water.
- Wash indoor fabric mats and curtains every 2 to 3 weeks or replace curtains and drapes with easy care wipe-down blinds.
- Increase air circulation. By keeping the air moving with fans in every room will remove stagnant air, the perfect environment for dust, mould and other allergens. Open all the windows at least twice a week.
- The use of an air purifier, though costly, does an excellent job of ridding most airborne pollutants.

PART FOUR

THE HANDS
EMOTIONS
BENEFITS

THE HANDS

The Australian Massage is an excellent therapeutic combination as the massage and the oils have mutually enhancing properties. Hand healing is the most ancient form of healing and so too is the application of oils. This dates right back in time to Jesus Christ when he received a foot rub with oils, and no doubt massage goes a long way beyond that time, more than likely before the beginning of the human race.

Fingertips are sensitive, finely tuned receptors. During The Australian Massage the hands learn what have most likely only been touched with your eyes, the geography of the human body. The hands become channels of healing energy. Not only do they help heal on a physical level they also assist in balancing on emotional and psychic levels.

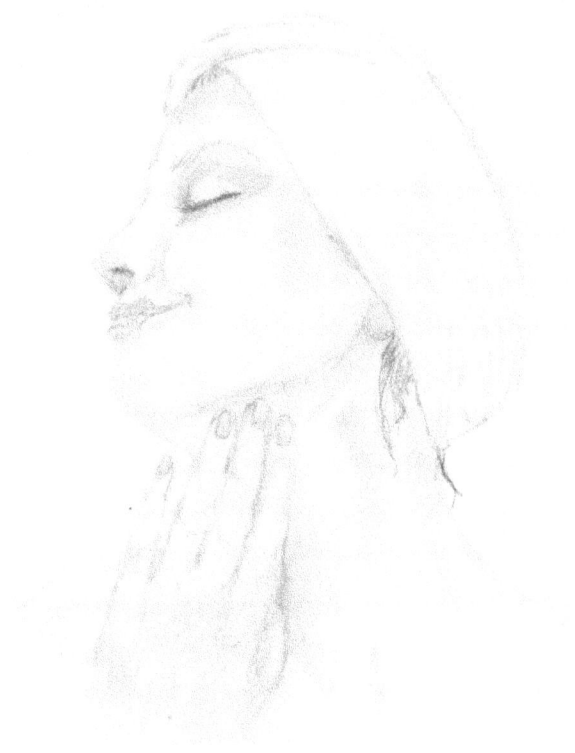

EMOTIONS

During The Australian Massage, it is not uncommon for the receiver to burst into fits of laughter, shed tears, or have a nose drip. The Australian Massage touches the deepest of hidden emotions. All of these reactions are natural healing processes in the body. Do not be distressed with the emotions, especially tears as these are both shed in joy and grief. The giving of yourself touches the receiver so deeply and is relieved at how much care you actually gave. In fact it is a compliment to the practitioner.

BENEFITS

Everybody can gain benefits from The Australian Massage in one form or another, even the practitioner applying it. Applying The Australian Massage is one of the most giving actions a practitioner can give. As warmth is projected into another this is giving healing support. The body needs warmth to survive. Warmth comes in many forms: the sun primarily, food, beverages, shelter and the breath, all are the most important factors in human life. What you project is what the other receives. The Australian Massage can give healing, healthy warmth from one to another, especially when you are a compassionate, empathising practitioner. If your hands are cold during the giving of The Australian Massage then you will need to listen to a positive body relaxation meditation to release blockages that are within your body before ever performing this healing method. If there are any past unreleased grievances, angers or resentments still being harboured within your body then these expressions too can come through your hands and be picked up by the receiver so make sure you are totally cleared from within of these emotions by tuning your ears to positive healing affirmations. Applying The Australian Massage with a cleansed subconscious mind is of utmost importance in giving your very best performance.

You may like to listen to my CD An Introduction to a Healthy Life daily until these affirmations begin to feel true for you.

The Australian Massage feels soothingly wonderful if given with a caring heart. When you are feeling 100% healthy The Australian Massage increases more bodily awareness, improving the senses. In times of extreme stress and crisis such as after the death of a loved one, miscarriage, any major change of address or within the home or change in career The Australian Massage is guaranteed to help you feel more balanced and better prepared to cope with these changes thus assisting with moving forward in life instead of staying stuck in the past.

As you learn you will experience total giving. It is natural if you feel some inhibitions when touching someone for the first time especially if it is the first application of The Australian Massage. After the first or second lesson this will diminish and you will look forward to each lesson as an exciting adventure. We both have a common goal and that is, at the end of this instruction book or/and DVD and CDs you have the knowledge and confidence to give healing to someone in need. If this is not so then you have more of your own emotional releasing to do.

Since nearly all physical contact has in the past been construed as potentially sexual, people avoid touching each other. A professional practitioner is high above this way of thinking. We know we are healthier with touch. Touch by consenting adults can bring immediate acceptance and unconditional love and when the adult body is suffering, whether that be emotional or physical, therapeutic massage can assist rapidly in the healing process. If you have any thoughts that are not for the receiver's highest good of her/his health then you need to clear away these thoughts and replace them with new healing positive ones. Listen daily to Pain Management & Preparation for Healing until you have clearly overcome them. You may even find you are healing other areas in your body and life that you were unaware of.

Do not carry a person's burden/s with you. During The Australian Massage the receiver will more than likely share personal stories with you. Leave them be. You are offering the best you know just by giving The Australian Massage. The right thing you can do for the receiver is listen. Reflect if you must. Listen, listen, listen and learn how to let it all go. Be grateful for your own health. Many practitioners find this difficult to do. Overcome this by listening to Daily Relaxation Meditation. The suggestions in this meditation will change any negative thoughts to healthy positive ones. A regular Daily Relaxation Meditation heals any negativity that you may have hung on to. Let it go every day. Develop the habit.

The Australian Massage which you are about to learn consists of therapeutic body massage techniques of the back, hips, legs, feet, arms, hands, neck, face and scalp. Upon completion of all the lessons The Australian Massage is performed in approximately forty-five minutes to one hour. With the addition of remedial work this extends to one and a half hours. Any massage treatment under forty-five minutes does not produce anywhere near the same therapeutic benefits.

Benefits of The Australian Massage:

- Induces natural relaxation unlike any other form
- Improves energy
- Brings vitality to skin
- Enhances sleep quality
- Improves concentration
- Better pulmonary function
- Improves the digestion
- Increases range of motion

- Promotes tissue regeneration
- Reduces scarring and adhesions
- Immediate circulation improvement
- Speeds up the healing process in body tissues after injury and surgery
- Aids in expulsion of stagnated toxic residue via the lymphatic system
- Decreases water retention and cramping associated with PMS

Performed functionally, The Australian Massage is also one of the healthiest massage methods available today when the body feels the need for a lift or a change. There is nothing quite like the magic of The Australian Massage to aid in letting go of the past and moving forward into the future with ease and serenity. With a caring practitioner it can assist in freeing the spirit of guilt, fear, anger, sadness or resentment. Continued research shows enormous benefits of touch ranging from treating chronic diseases, neurological disorders to injuries. Taking part in a regular self-care schedule may feel like pampering, however you may consider massage as a necessary part of your well-being plan. The more massage you receive by a caring practitioner the greater benefits you can reap. Your body will let you know when enough is enough. Always listen to your gut feeling. If you are the receiver always tell the practitioner of any moves that make you feel uneasy. If there is no change then sit up and voice your opinion. If you have and the practitioner continues doing the move/s you keep on sitting up and voicing your opinion until the move ceases or leave the premises making the point known to the manager, professional organisation or massage association.

When your body is in a constant physical state of 'stress' it moves through many changes: you breathe faster, digestion slows down, ulcers may develop, blood pressure increases, blood sugar changes, headache or migraine may occur.

The human body needs a peaceful and restful sleep nightly or daily to do its healing and restoration work naturally. If it does not receive this then it becomes distressed. Bodily distress also occurs if the body does not receive a balanced nutritional food and fluid intake. Daily enjoyable physical exercise, natural whole foods and beverages to fuel your wondrous body can maintain all of the systems in harmony.

When the body has become dis-eased The Australian Massage can induce deep relaxation, reducing stress, muscle tension, spasm and stiffness therefore joint flexibility increases, breathing is easier, circulation improves, the brain relaxes whilst also reducing blood pressure and easing headache. The internal organs function more easily therefore the body becomes more calm and balanced.

Along with The Australian Massage, according to Louise L. Hay, have a health check-up; go to the gym; walk; swim (enjoy water activities safely); dance; have some fun with your life; and work at a job you truly enjoy, one that uses all your creative talents and abilities, working with and for people who you love and that love you (Hay, 1984).

If you are living in a stressful environment such as having your couch or favourite chair close to or up against a wall that has a meter box directly on the other side of that wall it is of utmost importance to move the couch or chair two metres away from that wall to eliminate high electromagnetic fields (EMFs) emanating giving rise to additional stress.

ELECTROMAGNETIC FIELDS (EMFs)

Where you work is important. Electrical appliances connected to the mains will give off electric and magnetic fields when in use. Magnetic fields are generally measured in units of magnetic flux called microtesla in the UK and milligauss (mG) in Australia and America.

The Swedish Government has established a safety limit at 2.5mG. The Swedish standard is accepted throughout the world, meaning if someone consistently experiences exposure which exceeds their standard, that person could be at risk in developing health problems including leukaemia and cancer (NCRP Scientific Committee, 1995).

Currently there are no legally enforceable Australian standards regulating environmental exposures.

Because EMFs cannot be seen, the only way to determine if they are a problem is with relevant equipment and training (Bijlsma, 2010).

It is important to minimise EMFs where you spend long periods of time. According to Lucinda Grant (1997) a recent Electrical Sensitivity (ES) survey revealed the five most common symptoms experienced when EMF exposed were skin itch/rash/flushing/burning and/or tingling, confusion/poor concentration and/or memory loss, fatigue/weakness, headache, and chest pain/heart problems. Less common were nausea, panic attacks, insomnia, seizures, ear pain/ringing in the ears, feeling a vibration, paralysis, and dizziness.

The hormone melatonin helps the body repair cellular damage. It is produced by the pineal gland in the brain mainly at night. The pineal gland is "switched on" by dark conditions. EMFs reduce the effectiveness of melatonin (Powerwatch, 2012).

Reducing Exposure to EMFs

- Unplug or remove appliances that you don't use.
- Ensure you sit in your favourite chair at least one metre away from switched on appliances.
- Check areas where people spend most time that there are no major operating appliances on the other side of the wall, especially a meter box.
- Two pronged plugs are likely to emit high level electric fields.
- Avoid extension leads around a room.
- Bundle multiple cords together to reduce your exposure.
- Battery operated appliances are less likely to be an electromagnetic field source.
- Digital clocks emit high EMFs. Do not stand directly in front of an oven, dishwasher, or microwave.
- Keep at least one metre away from energy efficient fluorescent bulbs.
- Ensure the metre box is at least two metres away from the couch or your favourite chair or where a lot of time is spent.

For more information on electromagnetic fields you may like to look up Scientific Facts about Electromagnetic Radiation where it suggests that you don't stay under electric blankets (or on an electrically heated couch). Placing an electric blanket over a person while on a couch, as some day spas may do to keep the receiver warm during a body wrap is not recommended. For more information on this topic visit www.rainforestinfo.org.au/good_wood/emr_fact.htm.

To learn more about Building Biology™ see www.buildingbiology.com.au.

THE AUSTRALIAN MASSAGE MAINTAINS TWO GOLDEN RULES

- You must want to perform The Australian Massage
- The receiver must want to receive The Australian Massage by you

If these two factors are not met, it can induce:

- Stomach upsets
- Heart fibrillation/palpation
- Bruising
- Urinary tract infection

PRE-MASSAGE QUESTIONS

It is essential the receiver feels comfortable, secure and relaxed with you. A few pre-massage questions are asked of the receiver prior to commencement. A brief check before you begin brings peace of mind knowing whether you can safely give the person The Australian Massage, where to and where not to.

Q. "Are you taking medication for high blood pressure?"

A. "Yes."

The person obtains medical clearance from a medical practitioner prior to The Australian Massage. With approval, for optimum results, the application of the full therapeutic back and feet massage is recommended, maintaining very slow movements throughout, periodically observing the receiver's face for excess blood in the head. In the event of this happening, ask the receiver to roll onto the back and then you apply massage to both feet until the receiver's face resumes normal colour. Ensure all massage movements are performed very slowly.

Q. "Do you have a pacemaker fitted?"

A. "Yes."

The person obtains a written referral or you receive a verbal referral from the participant's medical practitioner.

Q. "Do you have any fresh injuries – i.e wounds, cuts, bruising, breakages, bleeding?"

A. "Yes."

Follow the St. John's or Red Cross or similar professional first aid instructions for injuries. The person obtains a referral from a medical practitioner. Do not apply The Australian Massage to any of these injuries until 48 hours has passed from the time of the injury and there are no signs of bleeding. If a person can lie comfortably, 20 minutes of gentle therapeutic back massage is most calming and soothing (i.e. if the injury is not on the back). Refer to The Australian Advanced & Metaphysicial Massage to release congested muscle fibres.

Q. *"Do you have varicose veins or do you bruise easily?"*

A. *"Yes."*

Do not apply direct pressure on raised veins, light effleurage only and always massage upwards or towards the heart. If the receiver bruises easily, apply no deep stimulatory movements anywhere.

Q. *"Are you 3 months or more into pregnancy?"*

A. *"Yes."*

Avoid all deep stimulatory massage movements to the lower lumbar, pelvic and abdominal regions (especially 3L – refer to the spinal vertebrae chart - Corresponding Areas of the Body Connected to Nerves from the Spinal Chord) and never have an over three months pregnant receiver laying front side down. Pregnant lady massage techniques are detailed and available in The Australian Advanced & Metaphysical Massage.

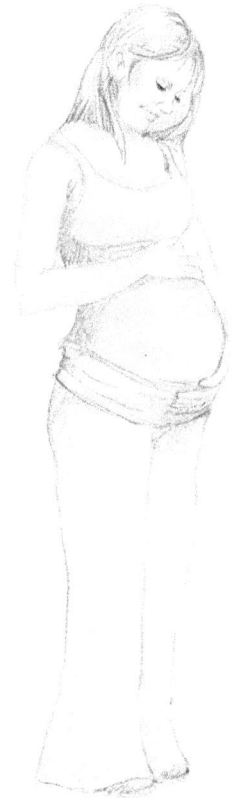

Are you sure this pressure is not too firm for you?

It feels a bit close to the bones!

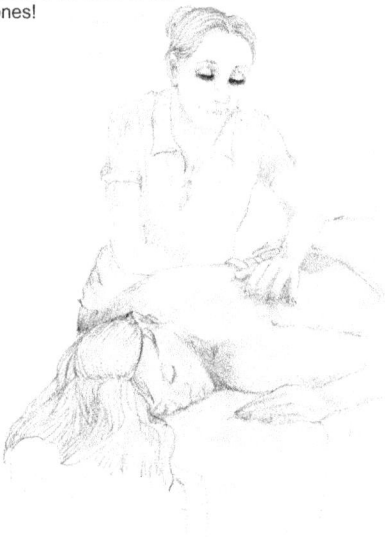

Q. *"Will you please tell me when the pressure is firm enough for you?"*

A. *"Yes."*

Q. *"You will let me know if you'd like the massage firmer or softer, won't you?"*

A. *"Yes."*

Q. *How's the pressure?*

PRIVACY

For all people and more importantly newcomers, it is essential the receiver feels comfortable before The Australian Massage commences. Allow time for the receiver to get ready. Make sure you are prepared and completely organised and the oil is warm. Have at least 3 other towels within easy reach. You may need to apply an extra one or two for maintaining warmth of the receiver and one rolled up for placing under ankles or anywhere else for extra bodily comfort.

Give the receiver privacy to change down to the undergarment and ask the receiver to wrap the large bath towel (that you prepared earlier) around their body. If you have disposable underwear the receiver may prefer to wear one of these, saving any oil coming in contact with the elastic of their own. Over time, oil tends to make elastic loose its stretch.

Disposable Underwear

and

Footwear

If you have disposable slippers, thongs or scuffs, provide a pair so that oil does not reach your floor when the receiver disembarks the couch, otherwise you will need to wipe their soles well with another clean cloth (warm and wet) to remove any excess oil so the receiver does not slip over and your floor remains oil free. Do not give pre-worn footwear unless totally sterilised. Always toss out worn disposables or give them to the receiver to have.

Let the receiver know you will return soon (as long as it takes to prepare your hands and oil). When you return ask if more time is needed before you enter. Ask the receiver if she/he minds oil in her/his hair. If so, place a hair cover/shower cap over the hair or a firm yet comfortable wide head band that holds the hair away from the neck, ears and face.

As the giver of The Australian Massage remain as silent as possible during the application. The more you talk the less your hands communicate and the receiver knows that she/he is not getting the most of what the purpose of why the receiver is there for, therapeutic massage.

You are a good listener for the receiver to speak to whenever the need arises. It is incredible how much you can learn in silence. Keep quiet and let your hands do the 'talking.' When you speak some of your energy disappears from your hands. Stay focused. If the receiver is speaking negativities play a positive affirmation CD so you both can benefit.

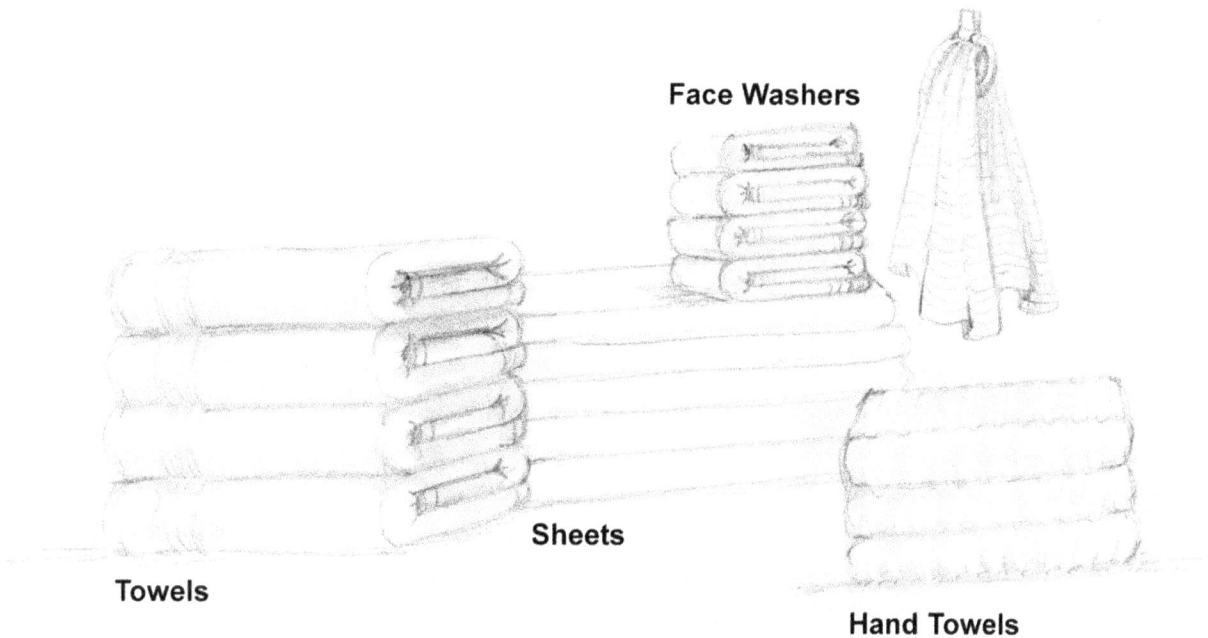

Face Washers

Sheets

Towels

Hand Towels

PART FIVE

BASIC MOVEMENTS

BASIC MOVEMENTS

Compression

A movement that uses control of energy is applied when making the initial contact with the receiver. This movement commences at the heel of the hand easing pressure towards the fingertips. The Australian Massage DVD shows how to perform of the following moves. Compression, a relatively new move (1993 resembles a rolling wave, very firm first, then easing to light before lift-off. It looks similar to an Hawaiian hand dance. The initial commencement was performed lightly to bring balance to the right and left sides of the brain.

The Soother or "Effleurage"

This movement is applied by using the full palms of both hands. Being one of the main movements in The Australian Massage, effleurage feels very soothing. The Soother is replaced throughout these instructions with the word "effleurage." The effleurage applied in Swedish Massage never originated in Sweden. It was called the Classic Massage. Johan Georg Merzger (1838-1909), a Dutch practitioner is the man who adopted French names to denote the basic strokes under which he systemized massage as we know it today as Swedish or Classic Massage (Calvert, 1987).

The term "effleurage" has been around for many years beyond my massage knowledge. As the move 'effleurage' is reasonably well known worldwide and more readily understood, this term is used throughout my instructions.

The Mover or "Petrissage"

The combination of lifting, rolling, pressing, squeezing and kneading are deep movements which stimulate the muscles and areas of fatty tissues, the top three layers of skin which stimulate collagen and elastin fibres, stretch muscles that have seized up and shortened either through injury or surgery, and relax contracted muscles from fear or over-extension. The Mover is replaced with the word "petrissage" (also used in Swedish massage) as this term is known amidst the massage industry and easily followed.

Palpation

This is a combination of small, firm, slow, circular movements which are very relaxing, almost hypnotic and transcendental. Palpate by using the balls of your fingers.

Friction

Friction is a combination of small, quick, firm movements that are applied using the balls of the fingertips to bring rapid nutrition to an area for more efficient healing.

Full Percussion or "Tapotment"

Tapotment is a term used when a combination of percussion movements are used. In the Full Percussion, the word "tapotment" is used throughout my instructions as this term is also known amidst the massage industry and easily followed. Tapotment consists of four separate actions:

- Cupping
- Flicking
- Chopping
- Pummelling

Cupping:

- Hold one hand in a hollowed mountainous peaked shape by bringing your thumb and index finger together.
- Bring remaining fingertips together, side by side.
- Straighten your fingers so that the fingernails are not pointing directly downwards.
- Hold the other hand flat and in a clapping motion, bring the shaped hand down onto it. If the sound you hear is hollow this is correct. If it sounds like slapping, then your peak is too flat. Make the peak higher. A hollow sound is always heard when cupping. Try cupping on your upper thigh muscles.

Flicking:

- Hold one hand vertical. Your fingers are held loosely together.
- Bring them down onto the other hand. How does it feel? If it stings your hand, lighten up until it feels good on your body. Try flicking on your upper thigh muscles. Now that you have your energy right for you, check with the receiver after applying two flicks, one with each hand. It may take some practice to have both hands balanced, giving out the same energy flow.

Chopping:

- Hold hands as for flicking, only this time stiffen your fingers and bring them down, one after the other. Test on yourself first. This move is used in The Australian Advanced and Metaphysical Massage on large muscle groups.

Pummelling:

- Hold hands in a fist shape.
- With thumbs facing you, bring hands down. Pre-test on yourself for energy output. Remember: the smaller the person, the less energy is used so be lighter in these movements. This move is used straight after "chopping" in The Australian Advanced and Metaphysical Massage also on large muscle groups.

PART SIX

BODY BASICS

BODY BASICS

Bones and Joints

The skeleton is divided into an average of 206 bones with joints where the bones intersect. Joints come in a variety of designs permitting bodily movement and most are held together by fibres called ligaments. There are some joints, like those connecting the skull's series of bones that allow no movement while others permit limited movement. Spinal joints allow some movement in several directions. The majority of joints have a widespread range of movement and these are known as synovial joints.

The bearing surface is smoothed by slippery cartilage reducing friction whereas the larger joints are lubricated with synovial fluid. Synovial joints are connections that are sturdy enough to hold the skeleton together permitting a range of motions. These joint ends are coated with cartilages to lessen friction and cushion against jolts.

A joint cavity is that narrow space located between the bones, giving freedom of movement. Ligaments position and control the bones. Mobile or synovial joints allow a wide range of movements that are lined with synovium oiling the joints, preventing them from drying up. Fibrous or fixed joints allow very limited movement by fibrous tissue such as those of the skull, sacrum, back, some ankle joints and pelvis where there is no synovium.

Synovial Joints

HINGE	Knee, Elbow, and Fingers
GLIDING	Spinal bones, Tarsal (ankle) bones, and Wrist
PIVOT	Neck (at base of the skull), Elbow (between the Humerus and the Ulna)
BALL AND SOCKET	Hip, and Shoulder
ARTICULATING CARTILAGE	Tough elastic material covering bone ends
JOINT CAPSULE	Tough gristle enclosing entire joint

| BURSAE | Contain synovial fluid and are located at joints where joint lubrication is necessary to allow movement |
| SYNOVIUM | Sacs lining the insides of the joint, oiling and lubricating it |

Bone

Bone is alive and consists of an outer layer: the periosteum, (outside skin of the bone); the next layer is hard compact bone and the inner layer is bone marrow. Inside it contains numerous layers. The first layer of thin, whitish skin is filled with nerves, blood vessels and supplies of cells which hard bone beneath is built.

The compact bone is very hard and shaped like a cylinder. Nerve and blood vessels supplying oxygen and nutrients to the bone run through thousands of miniature holes and passageways. The weight of the body is supported by this dense, rigid, cylindrical shaped bone that is made up mostly of calcium and minerals so that bone feels no pain. Because the skin is very sensitive, when the bone is broken, injured nerve fibres run through the compact bone and send messages relaying pain signals to the brain.

Surrounding and protecting the spongy bone marrow containing gelatine is the cylindrical portion of the bone. Marrow produces either red blood cells (to carry oxygen), white blood cells (to fight infection), or platelets (which help stop bleeding). The three bone layers work together with nerve signals swiftly moving back and forth and blood streams that move between the layers.

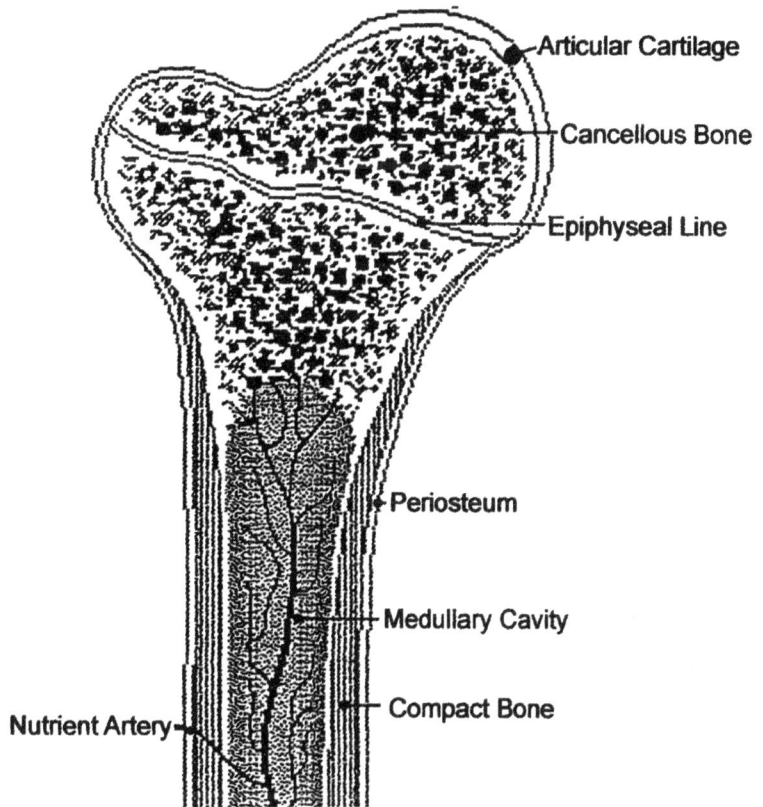

Muscle

You learned muscle co-ordination and control from your head down as a baby. First were your neck muscles, shoulders and arms, then your body, followed by the pelvis and finally, the legs.

Prime moving muscles such as the deltoids in the shoulders and upper arms are powerful initiators of force. Prime movers' contractions result in movement and are called agonists. Antagonists oppose their action; i.e. a muscle which extends a limb is acting against a muscle that flexes or bends. The antagonist is usually on the opposite side of a bone or joint in relation to the prime mover. The antagonist's action is opposite to that of the prime mover.

Assistant movers contribute a specific movement, often assisting the prime movers. In bending the knee the hamstring muscle of the thigh (back of upper leg) is the prime mover, the Sartorius muscle is the assistant, and the quadriceps are the antagonists.

What holds a bone or other part of your body steady to provide a foundation upon which your muscles can pull is a stabilizer. When lifting weights, the abdominal muscles contract to hold the hips and trunk therefore transferring momentum from the body to you when standing up.

A process that constantly loses and regains the balance is placing one foot in front of other as legs and arms work like levers, pivoting on fulcrums of ankles, shoulders and hips. Producing a rotary motion, propelling your body forward, upsetting the sense of balance are the legs.

The muscles synchronise movements of your arms and legs to ensure that balance is restored before the body topples over. Activities of fast and delicate natures and the movement of light objects are what the human body is best at. The human mind has designed tools and machines to gain a force advantage, compensating for the body's powerlessness to lift heavy objects.

Basic Skeletal Chart

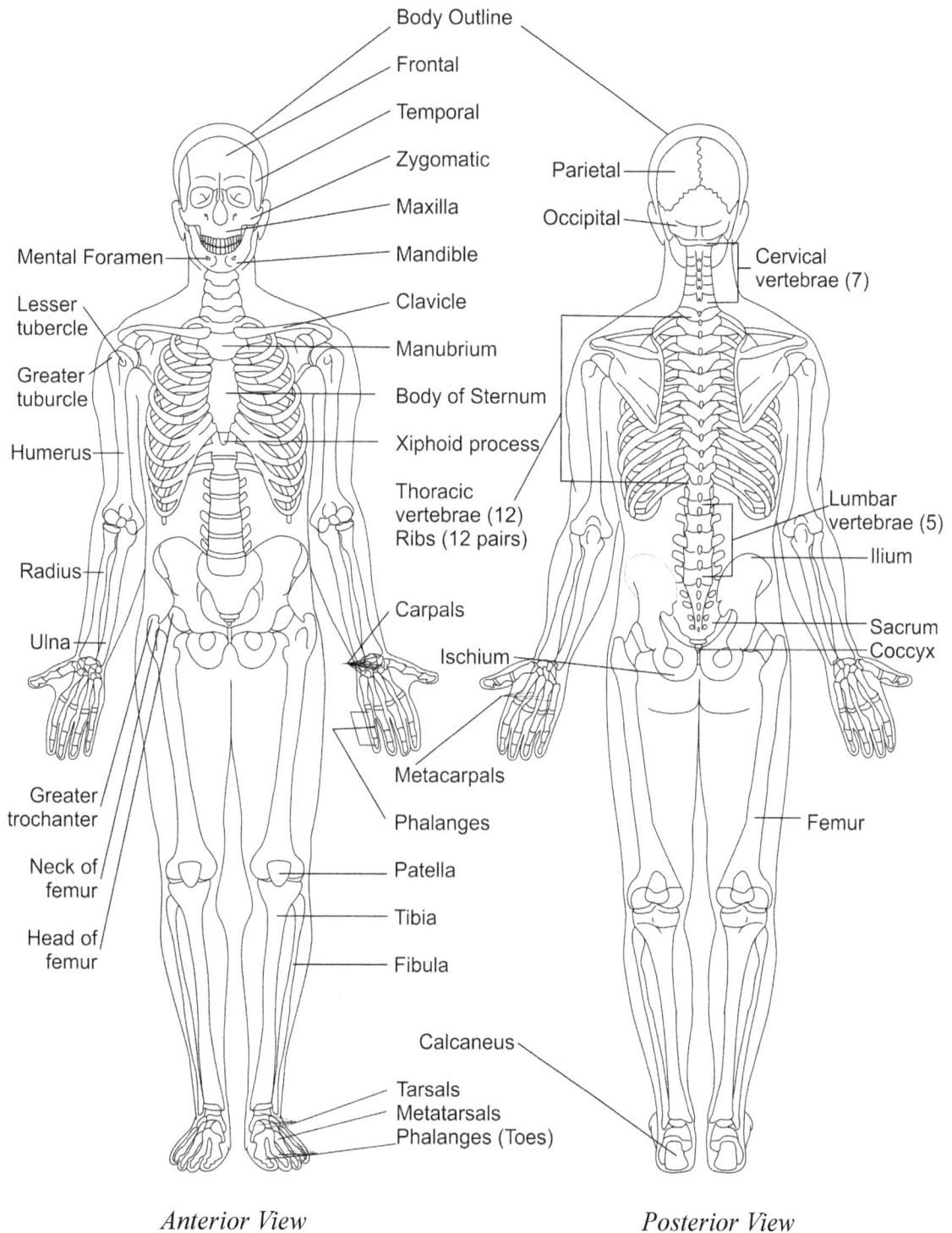

Body Outline
Frontal
Temporal
Zygomatic
Maxilla
Mandible
Parietal
Occipital
Mental Foramen
Lesser tubercle
Greater tuburcle
Humerus
Radius
Ulna
Clavicle
Manubrium
Body of Sternum
Xiphoid process
Thoracic vertebrae (12)
Ribs (12 pairs)
Carpals
Ischium
Metacarpals
Phalanges
Greater trochanter
Neck of femur
Head of femur
Patella
Tibia
Fibula
Cervical vertebrae (7)
Lumbar vertebrae (5)
Ilium
Sacrum
Coccyx
Femur
Calcaneus
Tarsals
Metatarsals
Phalanges (Toes)

Anterior View   *Posterior View*

Basic Muscular Chart

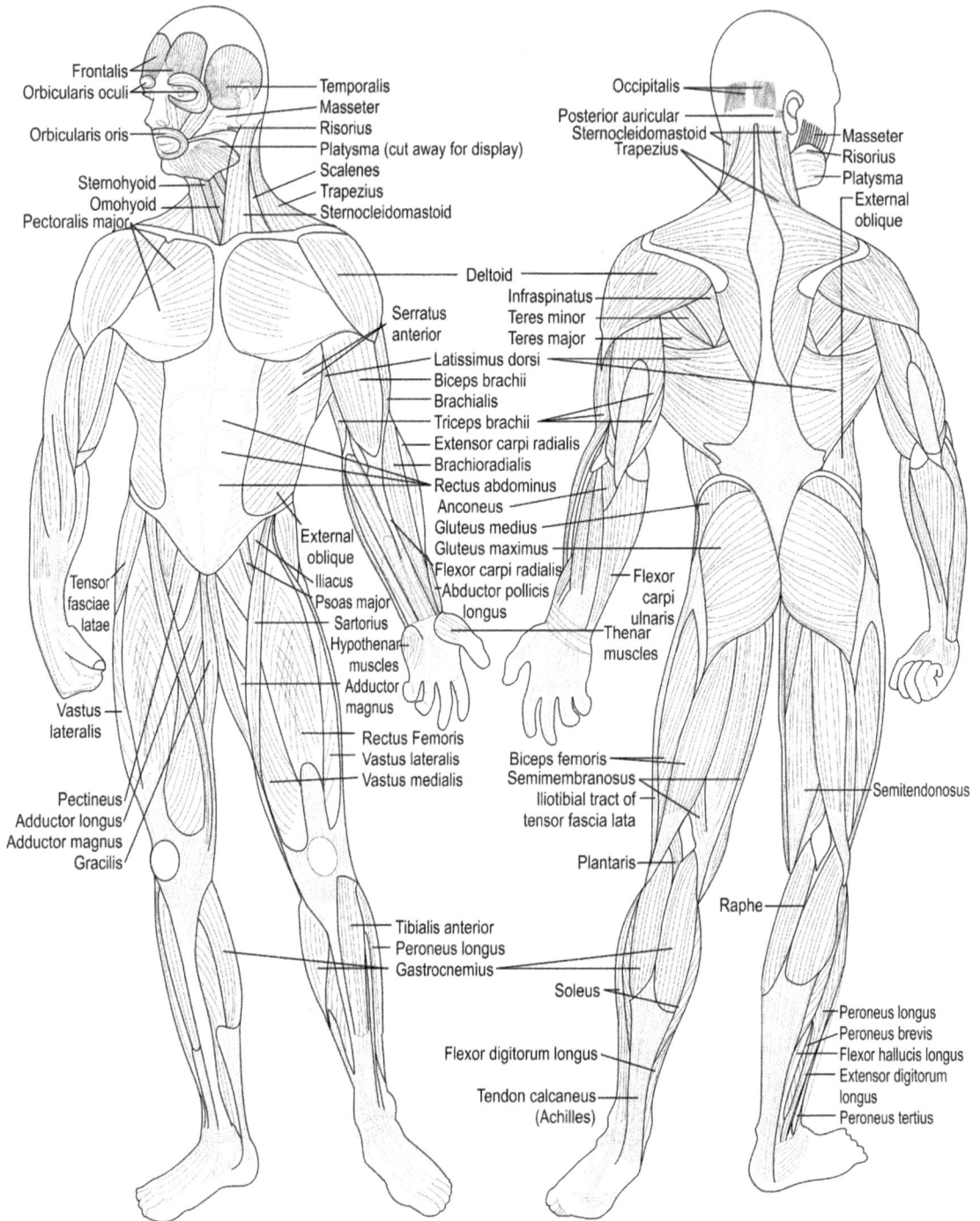

Frontalis
Orbicularis oculi
Orbicularis oris
Sternohyoid
Omohyoid
Pectoralis major

Temporalis
Masseter
Risorius
Platysma (cut away for display)
Scalenes
Trapezius
Sternocleidomastoid

Deltoid

Serratus
anterior

External
oblique
Iliacus
Psoas major
Sartorius
Hypothenar
muscles
Adductor
magnus

Tensor
fasciae
latae

Vastus
lateralis

Pectineus
Adductor longus
Adductor magnus
Gracilis

Latissimus dorsi
Biceps brachii
Brachialis
Triceps brachii
Extensor carpi radialis
Brachioradialis
Rectus abdominus
Anconeus
Gluteus medius
Gluteus maximus
Flexor carpi radialis
Abductor pollicis
longus

Rectus Femoris
Vastus lateralis
Vastus medialis

Tibialis anterior
Peroneus longus
Gastrocnemius

Flexor digitorum longus

Tendon calcaneus
(Achilles)

Anterior View

Occipitalis
Posterior auricular
Sternocleidomastoid
Trapezius

Masseter
Risorius
Platysma
External
oblique

Infraspinatus
Teres minor
Teres major

Flexor
carpi
ulnaris
Thenar
muscles

Biceps femoris
Semimembranosus
Iliotibial tract of
tensor fascia lata

Plantaris

Raphe

Soleus

Semitendonosus

Peroneus longus
Peroneus brevis
Flexor hallucis longus
Extensor digitorum
longus
Peroneus tertius

Posterior View

PART SEVEN

THE METHOD

CHAPTER ONE

THE AUSTRALIAN BACK MASSAGE
OIL APPLICATION

THE AUSTRALIAN BACK MASSAGE

Compression

Standing on the left side of the receiver, place the large towel over the back. Using the gradual full under-sided surface of both hands, place them firmly on the right side of the lower lumbar, right beside the spine, between the vertebrae and the longitudinal muscles of the spine.

Apply energy at the base of your palms. If you hear an expulsion of air from the receiver, lighten off.

Follow with the application of this compression along your palm. Commence at the heel of both hands, lighten the compression at the fingers, and then apply very little energy out of the fingertips as they gently float off the torso. This is the movement that looks similar to an Hawaiian hand dance. Continue with this compression movement right up to the top of the shoulder blade.

Maintaining physical contact, change sides by walking around the receiver's head. Repeat compression movement commencing on the left side of the lower lumbar. Firmness in this exercise is of utmost importance on an adult. Judge how much compression to apply as per size and physical condition of the receiver.

Compression prepares the receiver for your direct touch and it is this move which lets the receiver know just what type of massage is going to be performed. If you start with firmness but not too hard that it causes pain, you will gain the receiver's immediate confidence in your ability to be good at your movements and this will psychologically establish unconditional trust.

The feeling from your touch lets the receiver know where your 'heart' is and whether this person allows you to continue to be their future practitioner. These are your own feelings that move through your hands. If the receiver detects anger (very sharp and hard) or sadness (very soft and flimsy) through you, the receiver will more than likely go elsewhere.

This move also allows the body to commence letting go of emotions through the trust that has now developed. Whatever you do, never blurt out your own emotional problems in search of answers. Give yours to a professionally trained psychologist.

Towel Tuck Number 1

Lower the towel and tuck 2½cm (1") of the edge of the towel under the top of the garment. Check to see that the undergarment is not too tight. If it is, inform the receiver to wear easier fitting clothing next to the skin as this will aid in improving circulation.

OIL APPLICATION

You have now ready some massage oil, one that glides freely and lasts for many movements. If the weather is cold pre-heat 30 to 50mL of the oil in a bottle and rest it in a jug of hot water till it reaches skin temperature. Always check the temperature of the oil in your palm before applying to the receiver's skin.

Pour a small amount of oil into the palm of your left or right hand, never straight from the bottle onto the receiver. You must feel the oil first.

When the temperature of the oil feels nice and warm, apply commencing at the lower back. Glide straight up over the spine to the neck.

Use one hand to hold the bottle and the other to apply the oil from the bottle otherwise you will have an oily bottle and oil slicks everywhere the bottle sits hereafter. You will have enough laundering to do without creating extra cleaning.

Apply oil again at the lower spine. It is good to have a little pond of oil in the hollow of the back. Move your oiled hand out over the Deltoid muscle (upper outer arm), then up the spine again with more oil and out over the Deltoid ensuring plenty of coverage. Place the bottle close by and safely away from being easily bumped over or spilt.

Now using both hands spread the oil evenly over the entire back and upper shoulders, neck and sides of the torso. Ensure your hands glide freely over the receiver's skin. You do not want to pull and overstretch the skin at any time. Apply more oil when the receiver's skin has absorbed it thus ensuring smooth flowing massage movements.

BACK SOOTHER - EFFLEURAGE

Effleurage the back by using the full undersided surface of both hands, with fingers together. Place them on each side of the lower lumbar, pointing upwards towards the neck. Commence effleurage and slowly move up along each side of the spine.

Slowly glide both hands upwards simultaneously, covering the Trapezius muscle and the Sternocleidomastoid muscles on the back of the neck. Smoothly glide around the Deltoids at the upper arms, move down over the Latissimus Dorsi at the sides of the back, then returning palms to the Lumbardorsal Fascia at the lower back where you first started. Repeat this soothing move three (3) times.

Already the receiver is beginning to free tension from within the body. This rhythmic action is settling on the nervous system throughout the entire body. The brain sends out messages via the spinal cord into the nervous system that travels throughout the body.

When information received by the body's own computer (brain) does not match up with what either of the five senses (touch, smell, visual, hearing and taste) has learned previously, or knows instinctively, it reacts upon the nervous system and allows the brain to deal with this the best way it knows how. If the body doesn't react physically by way of doing some action to counteract the belief, the belief stays in the body. Unless the person learns differently, growths beyond normal bodily growth usually occur.

This is when it necessitates assistance and The Australian Massage is one of the best forms of treatment, reconfirming the love and care it so desperately seeks – touch – to reassure that life really is for living.

Positive affirmations listened and repeated through guided meditation or sung along to happy music are also very useful.

Back Soother

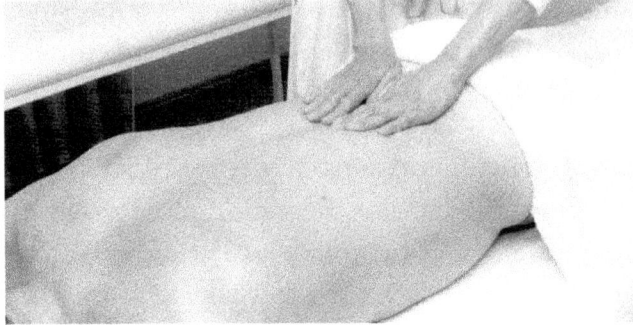

With towel secured into place, slowly move up each side of spine from lower lumbar

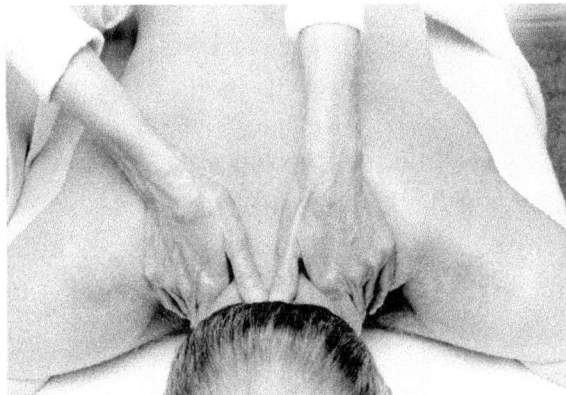

Effleurage into the neck

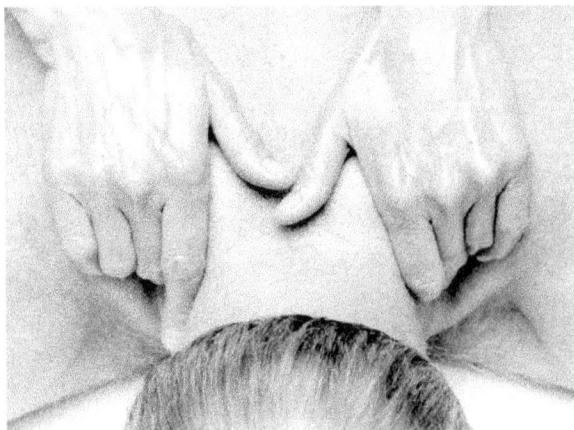

Effleurage continues from the neck

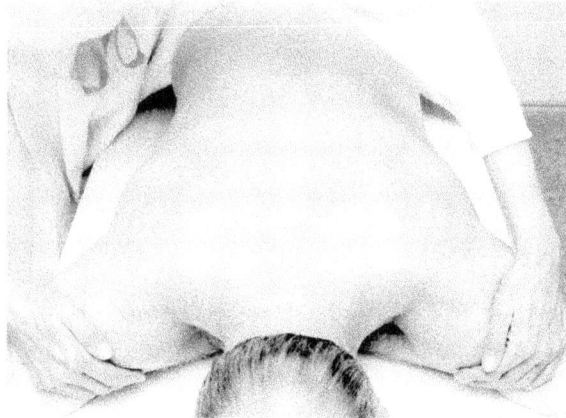

Glide out and around the Deltoids

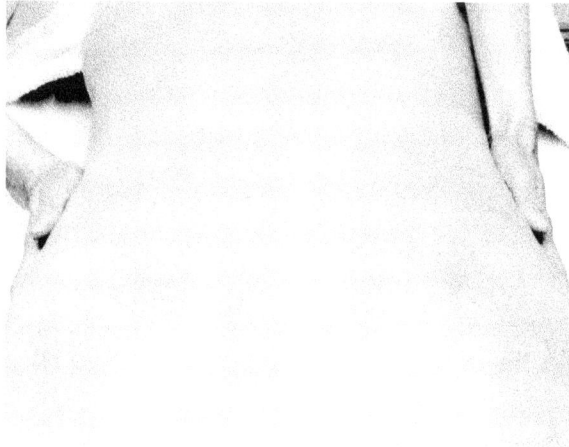

Continue effleurage down the sides of the torso, then return to the lower lumbar

GLIDE

Place your right hand on left and glide up along the left side of the spine to the top of the neck. Separate your hands and simultaneously glide across the top of the Trapezius muscle out to the shoulder. Repeat this gliding movement four times.

THE MOVER - PETRISSAGE

Glide straight into petrissage of the Trapezius muscle, all helping in releasing built-up burdens in the shoulders. Plunge your thumbs into the muscle above the shoulder blade as your fingers press into the Trapezius at the front of the shoulder, squeezing and lifting forward on a 45° angle to the torso.

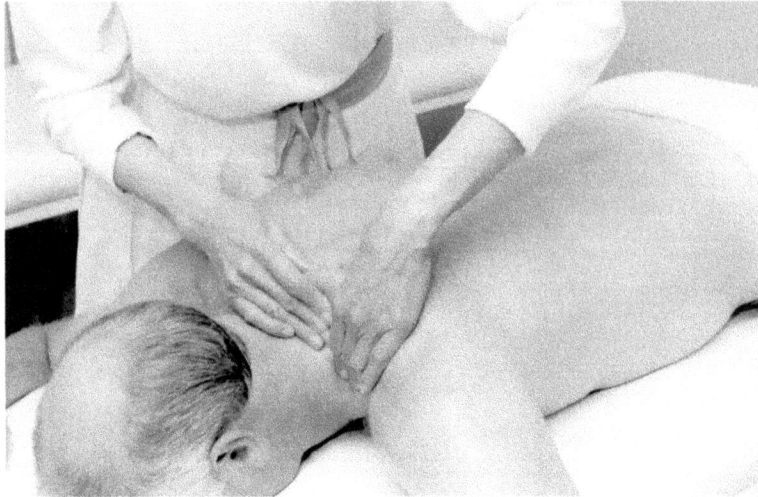

Petrissage the Trapezius

Change sides, maintaining contact, and commence gliding from the lower back with your left hand on right. Glide up along the muscles close to the spine to the top of the neck. Separate your hands and glide one hand after the other across the Trapezius muscle, out to the shoulder and flow into petrissage of the right Trapezius.

Standing now beside the receiver's head, with your thumb and index finger opened out, using only slight energy, very slowly glide up both sides of the neck to the base of the skull. Bring thumb and index finger steadily together, stopping just on each side of the spine respectively. Apply no pressure in the centre. Change sides and repeat.

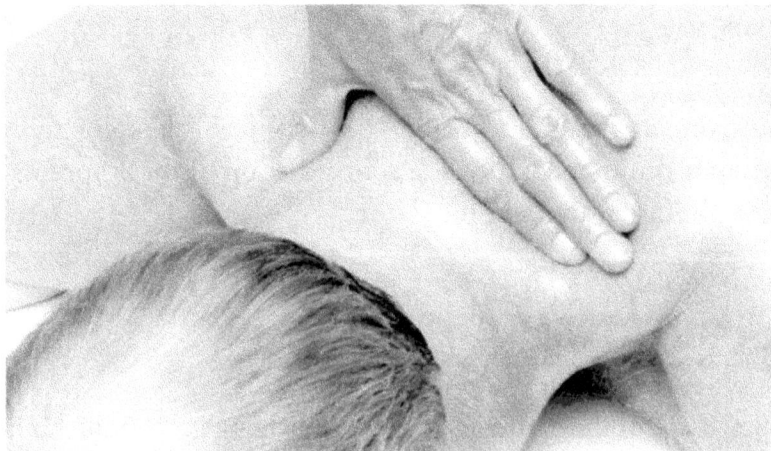

Glide up both sides of the neck

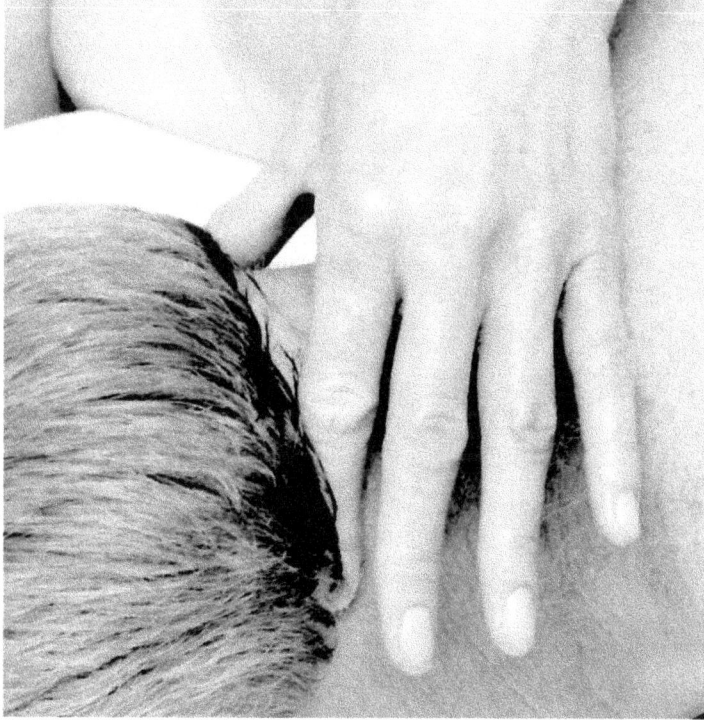

*Bring thumb and index finger slowly and
steadily together*

PALPATE

Stand in front of the receiver's head, facing the feet, and place the balls of your fingers (not the nails) at the base of the skull, staying clear of the centre of the spine.

Palpate the base of the skull, applying slight energy with your fingertips on the one spot without moving across the receiver's skin. The best direction to palpate is firstly upward and then out towards the receiver's ears. Remember to use slow, small, circular palpation movements. The right hand moves clockwise and the left hand moves anti-clockwise. All movements on the head are performed very slowly.

Extend closely held fingertips outwards, stopping just before the receiver's ears and palpate, right hand clockwise, left hand anti-clockwise.

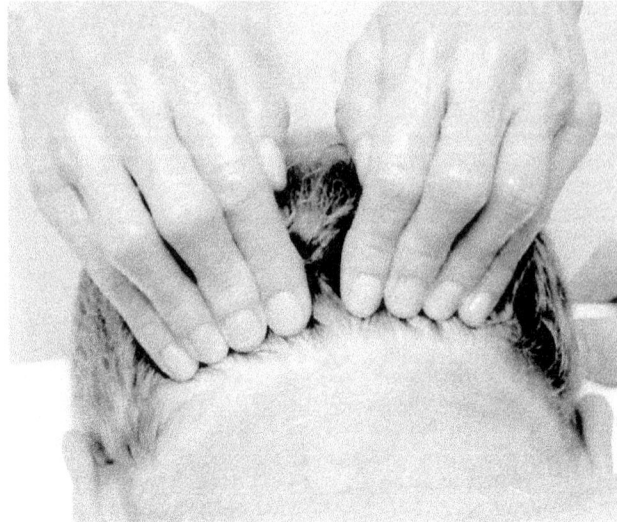

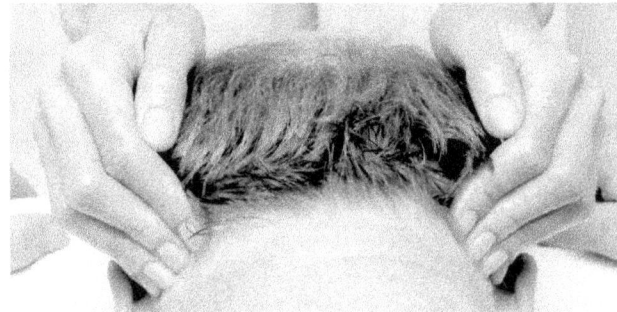

Place balls of fingers at base of skull and palpate using small, circular movements

Effleurage the back. Always effleurage after completing a specific movement. This gives a soothing finish after working on particular areas that may have given some discomfort to the receiver, through no fault of your own but old locked in tensions or traumas from past events held deep within the receiver's body that are now surfacing and leaving the body. This is the time when the receiver may want to talk, to open up and release the past, usually guilt, resentments or criticisms and allow it to leave the body permanently. This is when you listen, let it go and continue giving The Australian Massage. If the person does not talk this is fine. You may notice release areas rise to the surface leaving a red patch on the receiver's skin. This is good as now the circulation allows nutrition into the area to be healed.

With right hand on left, glide up the left side of the spine and palpate firmly into the muscles surrounding the Scapula (shoulder blade). Glide separated fingertips into the muscles. Feel your fingers freeing the muscle group surrounding the shoulder.

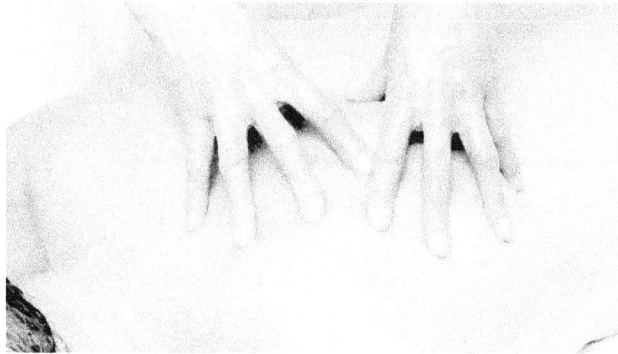

Palpate the shoulder

Now glide your thumbs, one at a time around the Acromion of Scapula, the bone joining the collar bone (Clavicle) to the shoulder blade. Repeat. Now palpate your thumbs down into the Deltoid 8 times, freeing any heaviness or obstructions in the upper arm muscle.

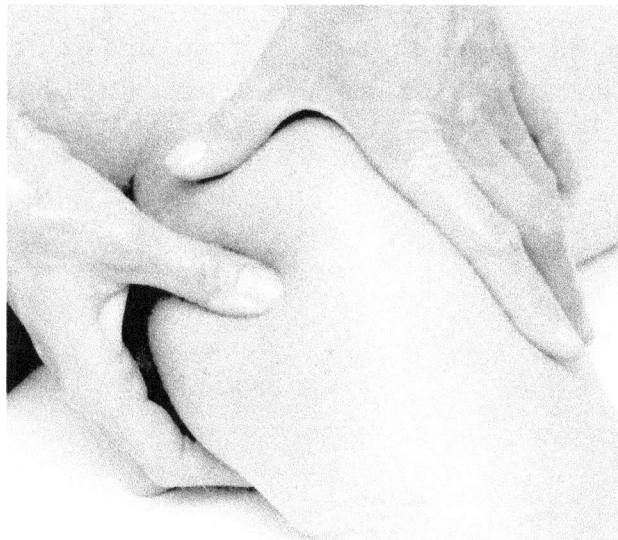

Glide thumbs around the Acromion
Palpate thumbs down into the Deltoid

Change sides and repeat. As you commence, your left hand is on the right side as you glide up the right side of the spine. Firmly palpate the shoulder muscles. Give an effleurage of the back.

TAPOTMENT

Cup and Flick the shoulders to no lower than the bottom of the Scapula (shoulder blade). Draw an invisible line at the bottom of the Scapula, from one side to the other so you will remember this and while you are learning pull the towel up to this line.

To perform cupping and flicking, stand with your feet wide apart so that you have easy access as you cup and flick without moving your feet. Using both hands, one after the other, with smooth rhythmic movements as you sway from your hips, commence cupping the shoulder on the muscles surrounding the Scapula.

If you are standing on the receiver's left side, always commence with your left hand. This applies for moves on either sides of the body:

□ Right side – right hand first
□ Left side – left hand first

With hands now peaked, allowing your feet to guide you, bring your left hand down. Follow with your right and continue cupping anti-clockwise around the Scapula, through the Trapezius in the neck, out over the Deltoids. Return to where you started, at the lower shoulder blade.

Tapotment is never applied below the Scapula (shoulder blade). This avoids upsetting the kidneys. Ask the receiver to inform you if your energy output is too heavy or too light.

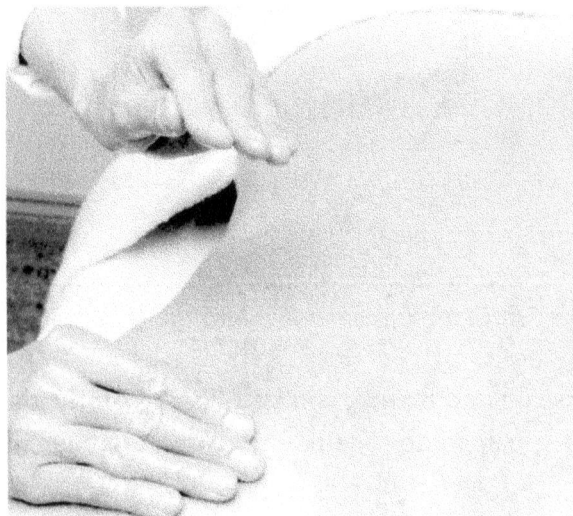

Cupping the right side – right hand first

Flow straight into flicking. Use loosely held fingers and brisk movements. Follow the same path where you cupped.

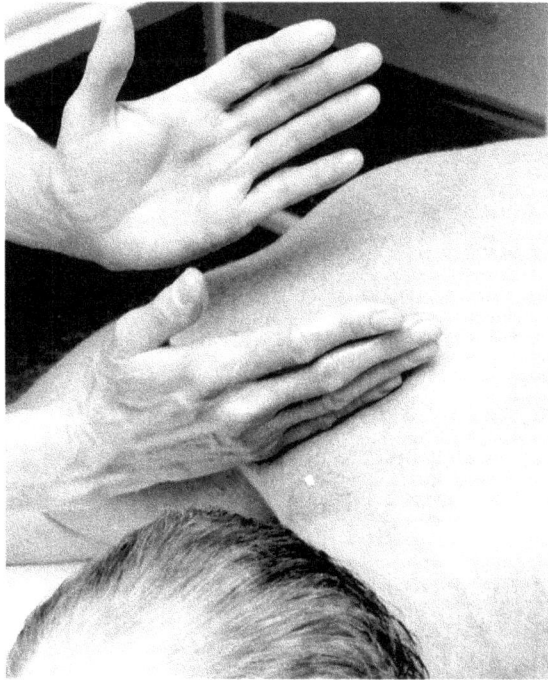

Flick the shoulder

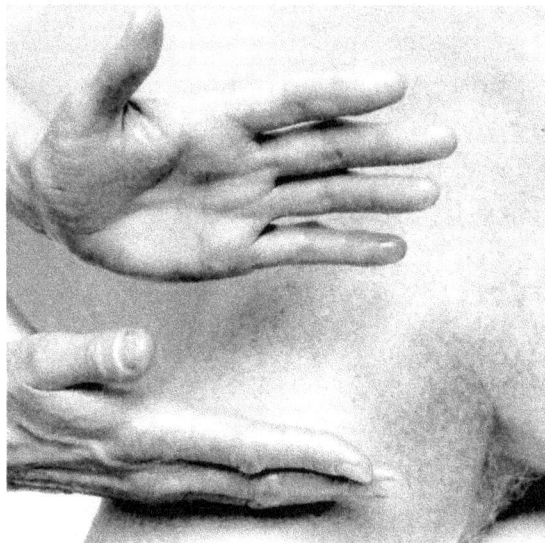

Flick the Deltoid

Smooth over the area where you applied cupping and flicking using anti-clockwise movements with the full palm of alternating hands.

SCAPULA CLEARANCE

Still standing on the left of the receiver, supporting the elbow with your right hand, bring the receiver's wrist around and gently rest it beside the torso at waist level. As the receiver relaxes, raise the shoulder with your left hand. With your right thumb and index finger opened widely apart, glide smoothly under the Scapula and upwards around it, separating the Scapula and Ribs. Bring your thumb right up through the Trapezius at the neck.

If the receiver's shoulder is not relaxed, either ask, "How much more can your relax your shoulder?" If this doesn't happen, place the hand at mid-centre of the lower back. This will enable the Scapula to fully relax. When you have finished clearing the Scapula, rest the arm by the receiver's side. (If you are applying this move to a member of the police force then I suggest this move is not to be performed without notifying the receiver as to what you are about to do. If you don't, you may find yourself with a lot of resistance and may even see the receiver upright, on the defence or ready to leave.)

Repeat the tapotment on the right side ensuring that both of your hands remain above the bottom of the Scapula (shoulder blade). Lighten your energy flow and effleurage the area. If the skin turns red in blotches or spots, then this is the receiver letting go of old inner tensions which is healing and healthy; that is unless you applied tapotment too heavy handed. Soothe over and separate between the Scapula and Ribs. Rest the right arm beside the torso. The receiver may prefer to place the arm down over the side of the couch. If so, ensure the arm and hand do not make contact with you. Effleurage the back.

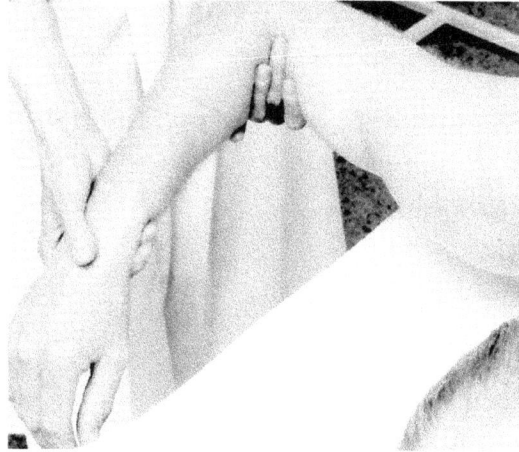

Supporting the elbow bring the wrist around

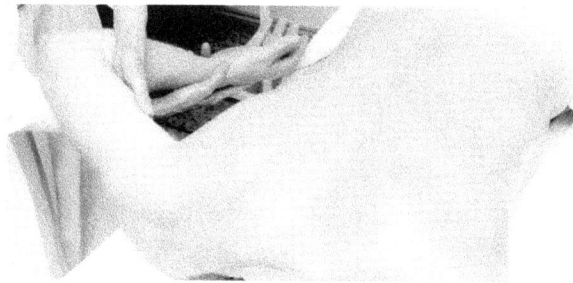

Rest wrist beside the torso at waist level

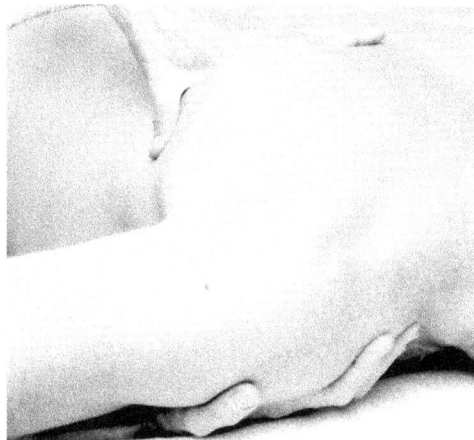

Raise shoulder. Smoothly glide under the Scapula

PALPATION ALONG THE SIDES OF THE SPINE

Commencing at the lower lumbar, using your right thumb and 2nd finger of your left hand, palpate up along the right side of the spine. Your thumb is pointed towards the 5th Lumbar vertebra. As it is pushed upwards with your 2nd finger, your thumb tip feels around each vertebra as it glides.

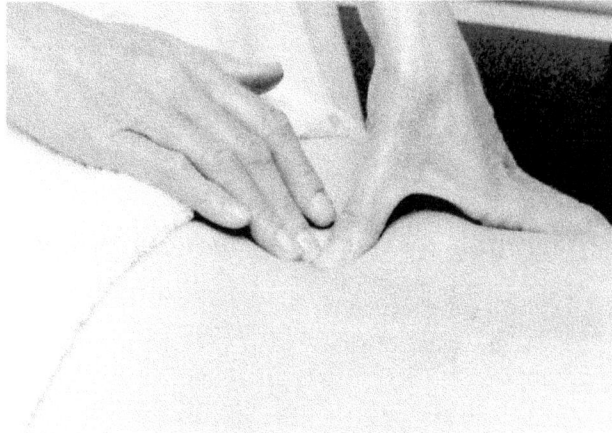

Thumb feels around each vertebra (on left side)

When your thumb reaches the 7th Cervical vertebra of the neck, raise your left hand. Continue moving your thumb slowly upwards. Place the heel of your left hand down on the 7th Cervical Vertebra. Now glide your left hand down along the right side of the spine as your thumb glides up along the sides of the remaining cervical vertebrae, to the base of the skull.

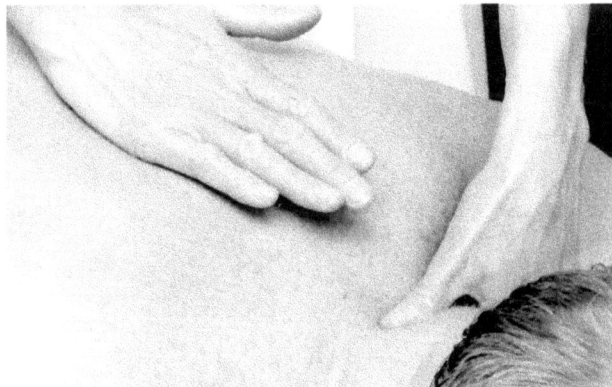

Glide hand down the left side of the spine. Thumb glides up along the left side of the vertebrae to the base of the skull

Maintaining contact, change sides. Repeat the procedure by palpating up along the left side of the spine using your left thumb and 2nd finger of your right hand.

Now stand facing the receiver's back. Commencing at the lower lumbar, palpate with your thumbs across the longitudinal muscles. Palpate, using both thumbs, one after the other across the right longitudinal muscles of the spine, up to the 7th Cervical vertebra of the neck. Now glide across the upper Trapezius muscle between the neck and shoulder. Change sides and repeat along the left side of the spine, allowing tensions to be freed.

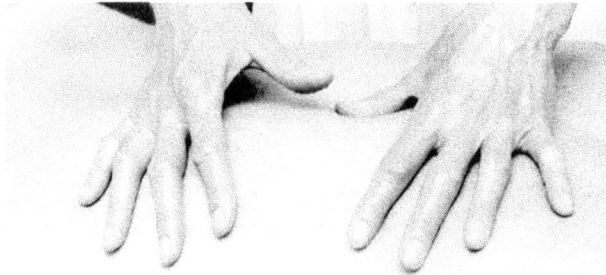

Palpate the longitudinal muscles (on right side of the spine)

FULL PALM ROLL

Using full palms, right hand first, roll across the back commencing from the right side of torso just above the outer hip, the Ilium, across the Lumbar, over to the left side and across to the Latissimus Dorsi. Lift gently off. Continue this move right up to the Trapezius muscle at the shoulders.

Change sides and repeat on the left side, starting with your left hand at the left Ilium. Roll full palms gracefully and firmly across the entire back. This feels ever so soothing, especially after working the spine.

RIBS SEPARATION

Separate the right ribs by bringing your left hand onto your right hand. Glide up from the right lower lumbar until you reach the bottom of the Scapula. Now turn your hands downwards and glide slightly separated fingertips between each rib below the Scapula.

Maintaining contact, change sides. Separate the left ribs by placing your right hand on your left hand. Glide up along the left side of the spine to the bottom of the Scapula, using firm, smooth, flowing movements through the Intercostal muscles of the ribs, relaxing the internal organs which the ribs protect.

When the Intercostal muscles are tensed, the ribs close in placing from light to moderate or enormous pressure on the internal organs. This tension creates tightness on the lungs, bodily discomfort, and pain. The back massage eases pressure allowing the body to return to feeling relaxed and more comfortable. Effleurage the back.

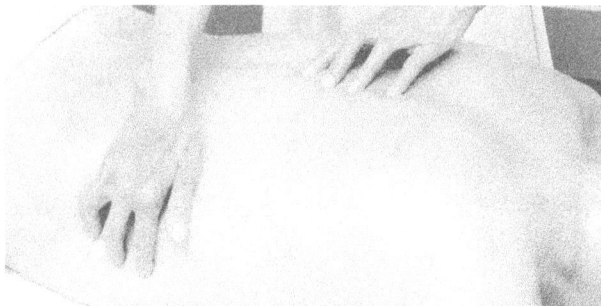

Glide separated fingertips between each rib below the Scapula

FIGURE 8 OF THE BACK AND DELTOIDS

If standing on the right side of receiver, with right hand on left, glide firmly up along the left side of the spine to the top of the shoulder (and vice versa if standing on the left side). Continue out and around the Deltoid (upper arm), down over the Latissimus Dorsi (upper side of the torso), External Oblique (lower side of torso) to the Ilium, and over the Thoracolumbar Fascia at the lower spine. Now your hands are on the same side as you are standing. Direct your hands upwards and glide up the right side of the spine, into the Trapezius, out and around the Deltoid, down the side of the torso to the hip, and then across to the 5th Lumbar Vertebra.

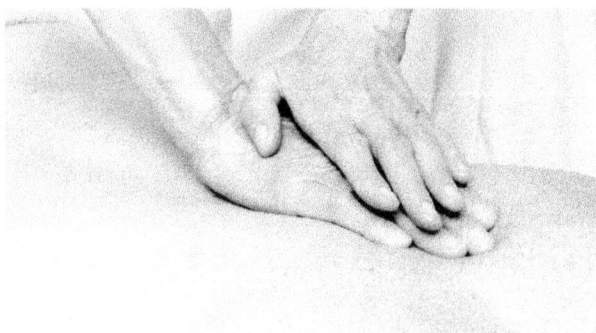

Glide up the side of the spine

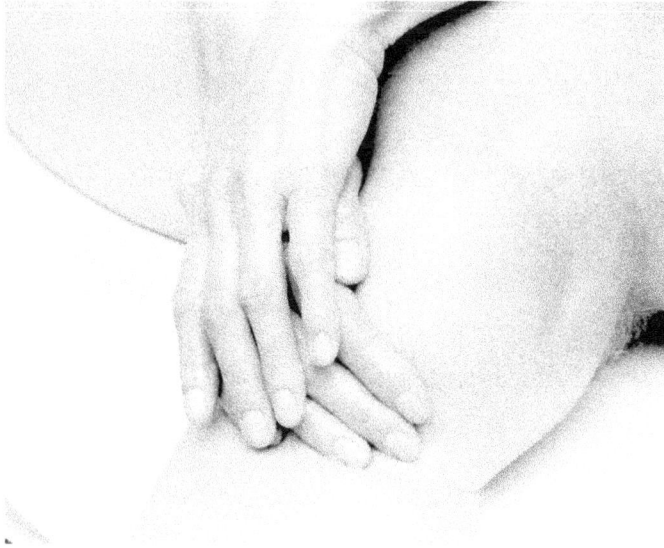

Figure 8 around the Deltoid

Separate your hands. Place your left hand on the left side of the lumbar, right hand on the right side on the lumbar. Now give a firm effleurage of the back.

Commence another effleurage. As your hands reach the Trapezius muscle at the shoulders, branch out to the Deltoids with ultra-smoothness and gently lift your hands off.

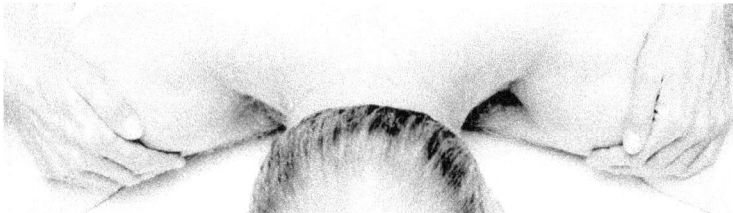

Branch out to the Deltoids

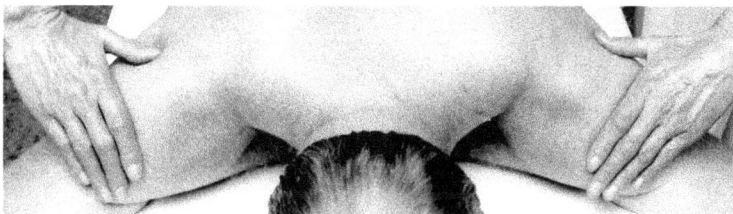

Gently lift hands off

CHAPTER TWO

THE BACK OF THE LEGS

THE BACK OF THE LEGS

Towel Tuck Number 2

Move the towel from the original position and place across and over the back and buttocks (Gluteals). The lower edge of the towel is now down to the knees.

Stand on the right side of the receiver. With your left thumb and index finger, grasp the bottom of the towel, between the receiver's knees ensuring you do not touch the inner thighs. Now with your right hand, hold the upper left side of the towel closest to the torso.

Pull the towel line between both hands straight and tightly across to the receiver's right side. The lower edge of the towel is now shaped like a half " V " i.e. " \ " from the knee to the side of the torso. Now bring the top of the towel in towards the centre of the back, neatly resting it there. The lower edges of the towel are now in a " V " shape at the sides of the undergarment.

Tuck 2½ cm (1") of towel edge under the top of the undergarment to protect it from oil. You now have full access to work comfortably on the legs. With this towel tuck, it will remain in place for the entire leg massage, giving you full access to the leg.

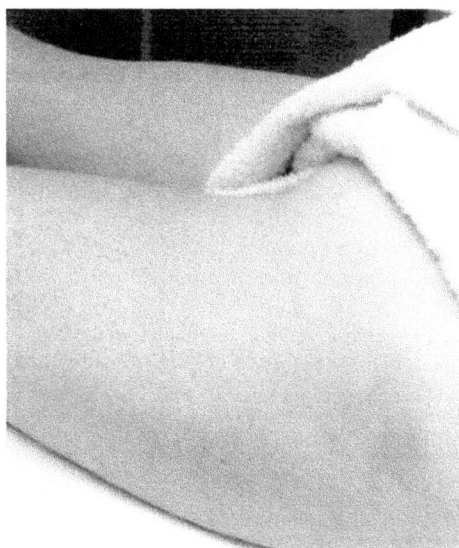

Towel Tuck Number 2

Oil Application

If the room is warm you can apply oil to both legs. If it is cool, only apply oil to the leg you are about to work on and cover the other leg with another towel.

Commencing at the upper leg (hamstrings) oil the leg down to the ankle. Do not apply oil to the soles of the feet. There will be enough oil on the legs that will smooth onto them during effleurages. Only apply oil to the heels if they are cracked and dry.

UPPER LEG

Effleurage the right leg. Place your right hand on left, fingers together and pointed towards your wrists. Commence effleurage with hands held in the " / " shape above the knee. With firm pressure, glide your hands up to the towel. Now separate your hands.

Covering as much of the leg as possible, glide lightly down the entire leg. When you reach the ankle, the left palm glides into the arch of the foot and the right hand glides over the front of the foot, and gently gliding off at the toes.

Repeat the effleurage 2 times, commencing above the knees at the hamstrings. Glide up to the Tensor Fasciae Latae muscle. Separate your hands and effleurage down over the thigh, lower leg, ankle, foot and off at the toes.

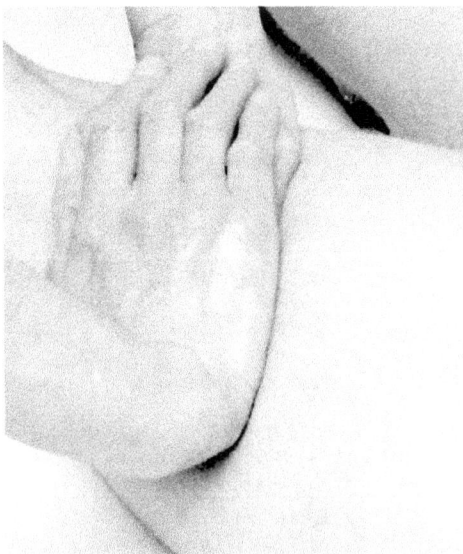

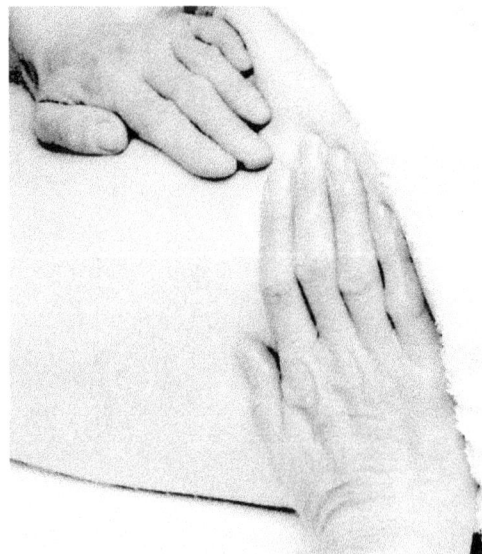

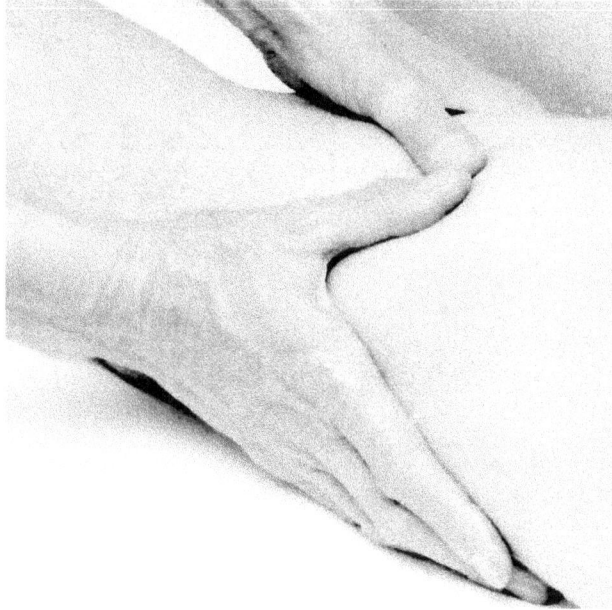

Effleurage leg with hands in "/" shape. Separate hands, and effleurage down the leg

Commencing with your right hand, glide fingertips around the Greater Trochanter at the top of the outer leg (the protruding bone). Now glide around the Greater Trochanter and into the Head of the Femur with your left fingertips. Repeat this move 3 times.

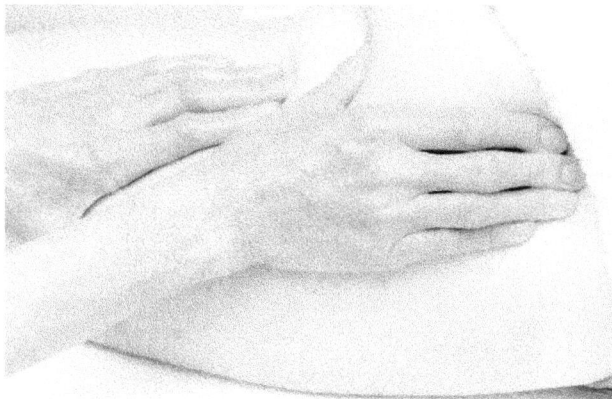

Glide around the Greater Trochanter into the Head of the Femur

Petrissage the hamstring muscles on the back of the upper leg, Tensor Fasciae Latae and Vastus Lateralis muscles, avoiding any varicose veins.

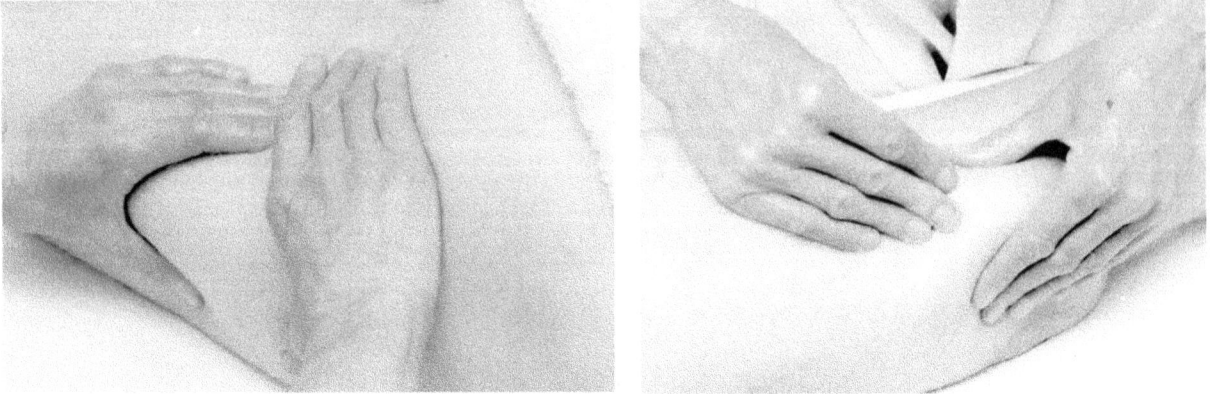

Petrissage the hamstrings

Move the petrissage down, commencing at the outer leg (Tensor Fasciae Latae), into the Biceps Femoris, Semitendinosus and Semimembranosus, and Gracilis muscles.

Cup the upper leg, avoiding the back of the knee. Flick, then effleurage the hamstrings.

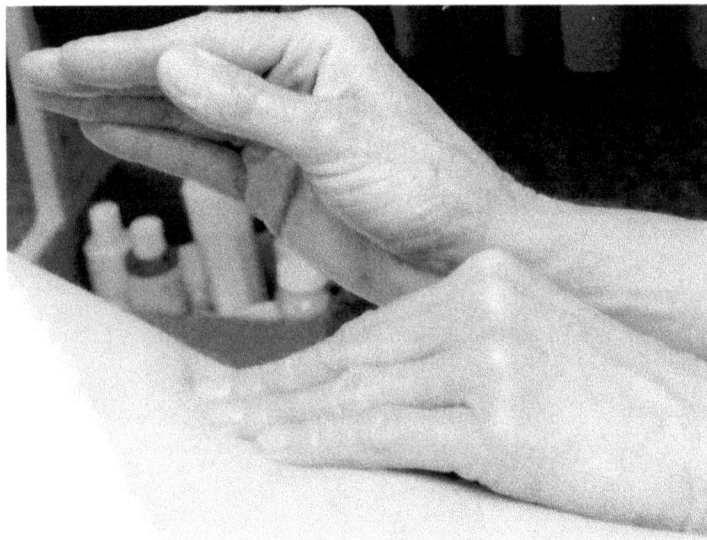

Cup the upper leg

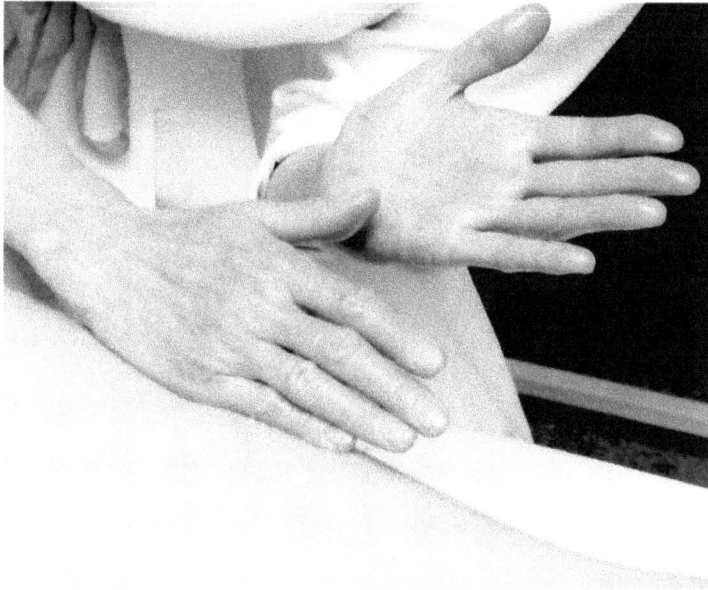

Flick the upper leg

LOWER LEG

Petrissage the Gastrocnemius muscle (calf or major lower leg muscle). Separate it slightly on the way up the leg and petrissage on the way down towards the ankle.

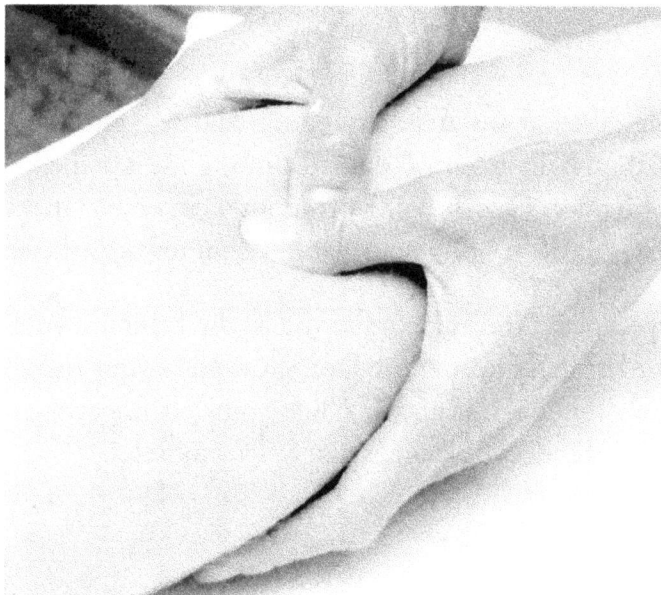

Separate the Gastrocnemius

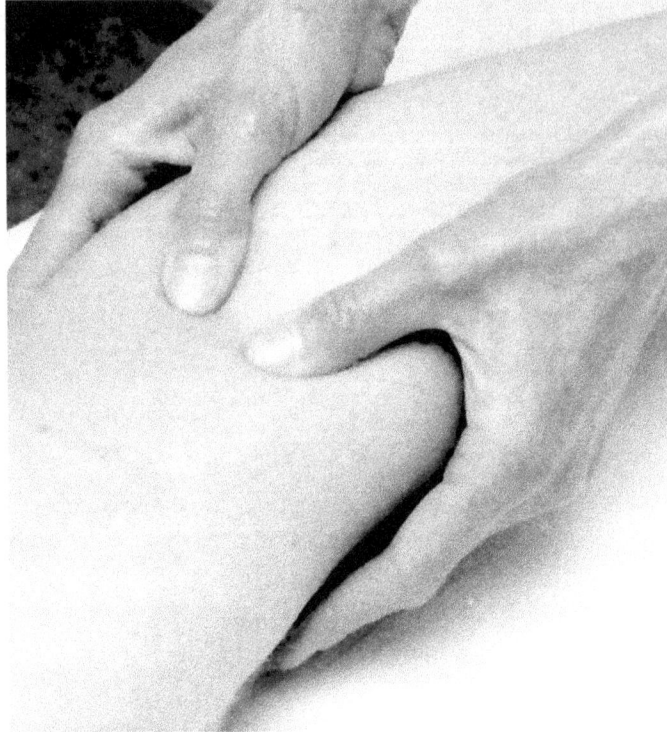

Petrissage down the lower leg

Petrissage the Soleus muscle, remember to avoid any varicose veins. Cup the Gastrocnemius muscle with peaked hands. Ensure that your cupping has the hollowed sound. Now flick the lower leg and effleurage.

Effleurage the entire leg. Turn at the Achilles Tendon and separate the Gastrocnemius muscle (calf). With your left thumb in front of right thumb, glide up the centre of the lower leg, starting at the Achilles (Tendon Calcaneus). Stop about 4 cm or 1 ½ inches before you reach the back of the knee. Petrissage as you bring your hands down towards the ankle. Repeat 3 times.

Effleurage the leg. As you reach the ankle, raise the leg by bringing your right hand under the ankle. Follow with your left hand raising the foot. Now glide your right fingertips firmly down along the left side of the Tendon Calcaneus. Glide your left fingertips firmly down along the right side and separate the Tendon Calcaneus and Soleus muscles.

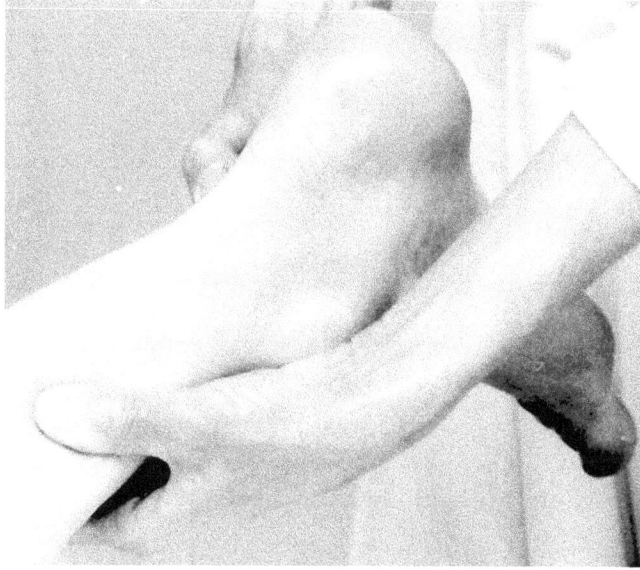

Glide fingertips firmly down the sides of the Tendon Calcaneus

Effleurage the front lower leg. Gently lower the foot. Palpate the Tarsals (ankle bones) in a clockwise direction, round and round, using your fingertips of both hands simultaneously.

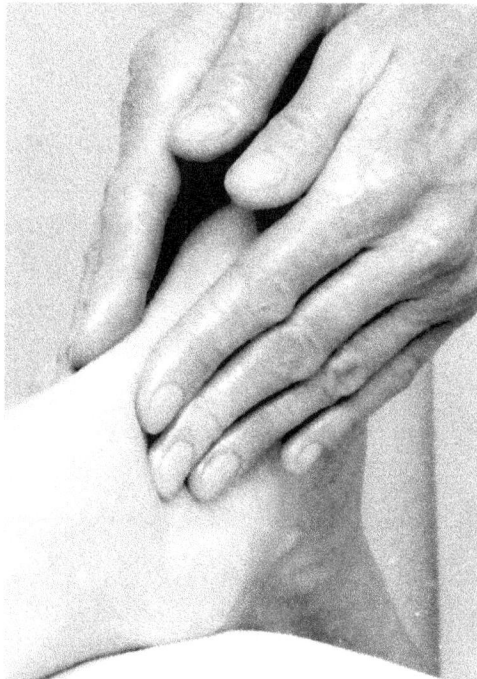

Palpate the Tarsals (ankle bones) in a clockwise direction

FOOT

Effleurage the foot, raising it slightly to do so. Turn and face across the receiver's foot. Raise the right foot and hold it at the ankle with your left hand. Make a fist with your right hand. Give a Figure 8 on the sole of the foot. Commencing at the heel, follow along the left side of the sole as it faces you. Veer to the right just before the toes. Turn. Move down towards the left side of the heel. Complete this move in the shape of a Figure 8 on the sole of the foot.

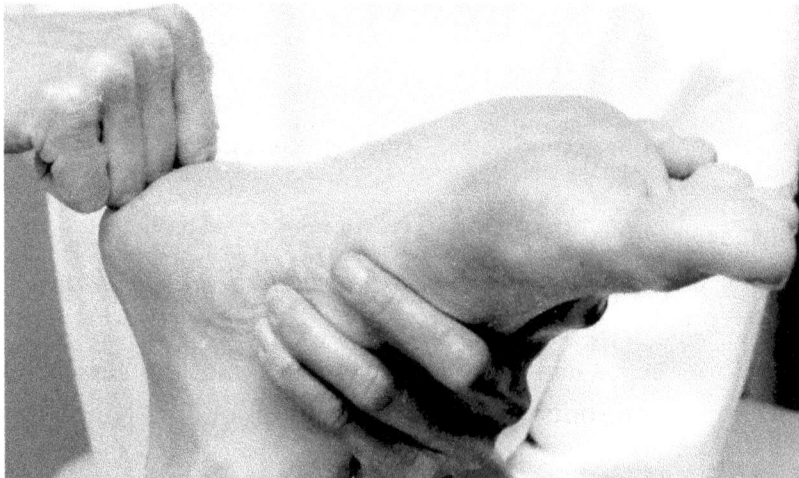

Make a fist and give a Figure 8

Repeat the Figure 8 on the sole of the foot. Start at the Calcaneus (heel). Follow out to under ankle, across and into the arch of the foot in front of the heel, out to the outer side of foot leading to the little toe. Turn right. Cross between the 2nd, 3rd and 4th toes. Turn towards the ankle, crossing at the arch, and return to the Calcaneus. This looks like a Figure 8 applied to the sole of the foot using your knuckles.

Flick the sole with your right hand as your left hand holds and supports the ankle and toes. Effleurage the sole with your right palm commencing at the Calcaneus and off at the toes (phalanges).

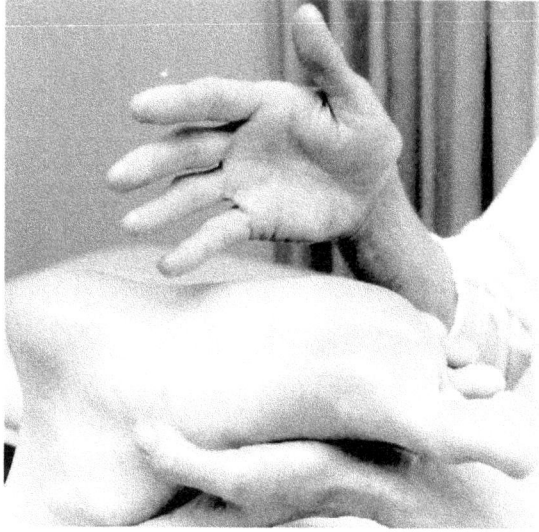

Flick the sole

METATARSAL SEPARATION

Sit on the lower end of the couch facing the receiver's head. You deserve to take the weight off your feet for a few brief moments. With foot still raised, separate the Metatarsals (long bones of the foot).

Place your left thumb on the largest knuckle of the big toe and your right thumb on the next toe's largest knuckle. Place your fingertips on the sole between the big toe and the next. Pull your right fingers towards you as you push your left thumb forward. Now pull your left fingers towards you as you push away with your right thumb. Continue separating the Metatarsals along to the little toe.

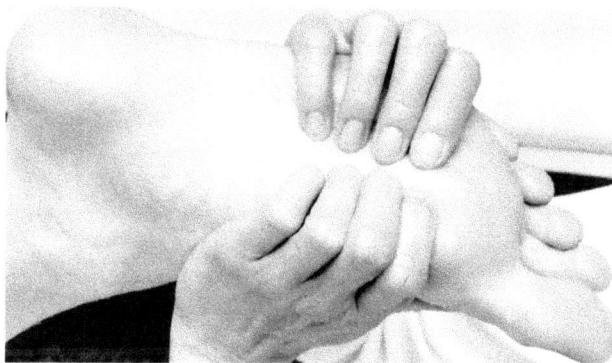

Separate the Metatarsals

Supporting the foot in your left hand, roll your thumb between the Metatarsals. Effleurage the foot. Effleurage the entire right leg and foot.

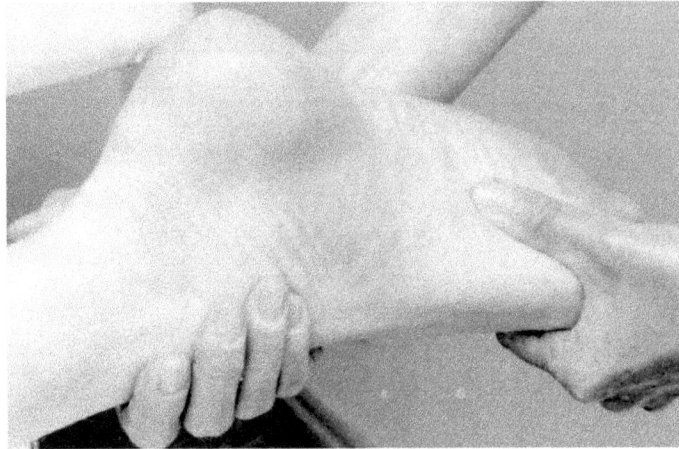

Effleurage the foot (1)

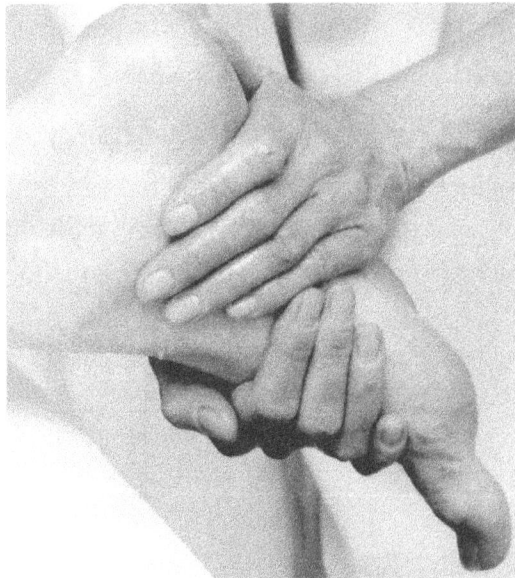

Effleurage the foot (2)

SCIATIC LIFT

Upon completion of the left leg, effleurage the right leg, then bring both legs together at the ankles. Place your left hand on the outer left thigh and right hand on the outer right thigh. Firmly glide up from above the outer knees into the top of the Femur (thigh bone). Squeeze the heel of your hands in and lift upwards, raising the sciatic nerve, releasing any built-up pressure.

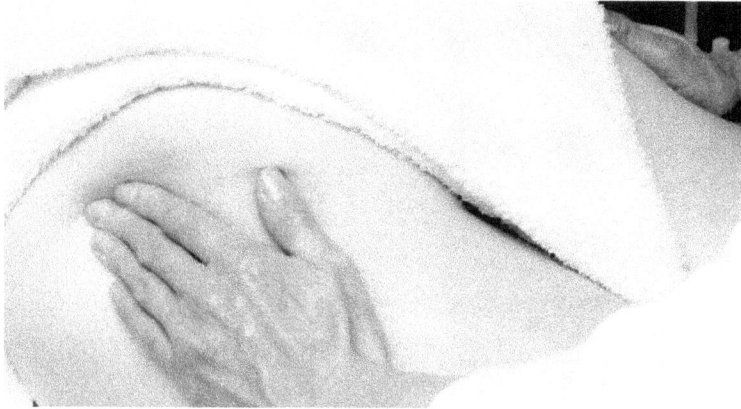

Glide up from above outer knees into the top of the Femur

BACK COMPLETION

Remove the towel from around the undergarment, making sure the receiver feels comfortable, and place the towel in position as for The Australian Back Massage.

Add a few drops of oil to your hands and apply Figure 8 movements of the back. As your hands return to the lower lumbar, separate your hands. Branch into an effleurage. Finish smoothly and lightly off the Deltoids.

Place the towel over the entire back, ensuring the towel is covering the receiver from the shoulders above the armpit down to the knees. Spread more of the towel on the other side of the couch. Lean your weight, pressing the towel to the couch, closest to you. Using both hands, hold onto the other side of the towel that is on the side of the couch at the top and bottom. Raise it to the height of the receiver's back.

Correct towel positioning gives complete privacy to the receiver. The receiver is under no misconceptions as to the Holistic benefits of The Australian Massage. Now ask the receiver to roll away from you onto the back keeping the torso completely covered during this entire procedure.

CHAPTER THREE

ARMS, WRISTS,HANDS AND SHOULDERS

ARMS, WRISTS,HANDS AND SHOULDERS

The receiver is on the couch with head now resting above the face hole. This allows for freedom of your moves between the back of the neck and upper Trapezius. The receiver's torso is covered down to the knees. Place the arms on the outside of the towel if the receiver is warm. If the room is warm you can apply oil to the shoulders, arms and hands. If it is cool, only apply oil to the left shoulder, arm and hand you are about to work on and leave the other arm covered with the towel. Check to see if the receiver is warm enough. By now, you may need to cover the legs and feet with another towel. Most people become very cool during or at the end of The Australian Massage because the metabolism slows during the massage.

UPPER ARM

With left hand on right, effleurage the right arm. Commence with your right hand over the top of the shoulder. Effleurage down the entire arm, and gently flow off the fingertips. Repeat effleurage 3 times.

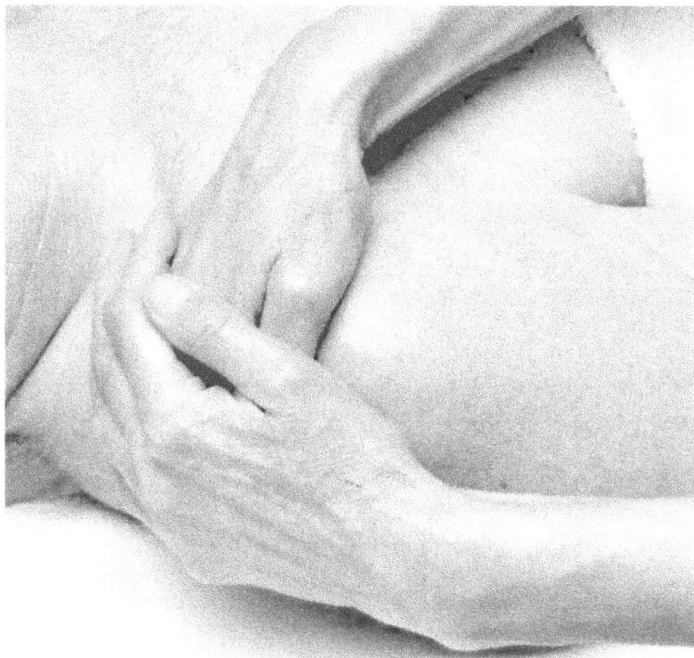

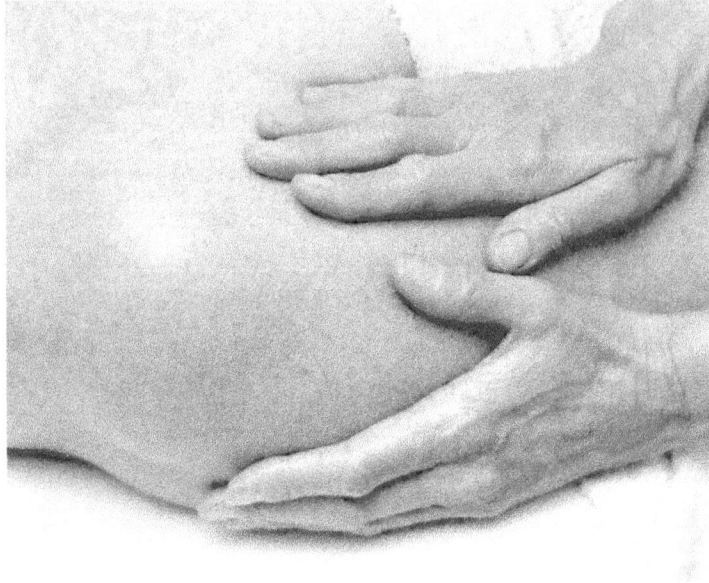

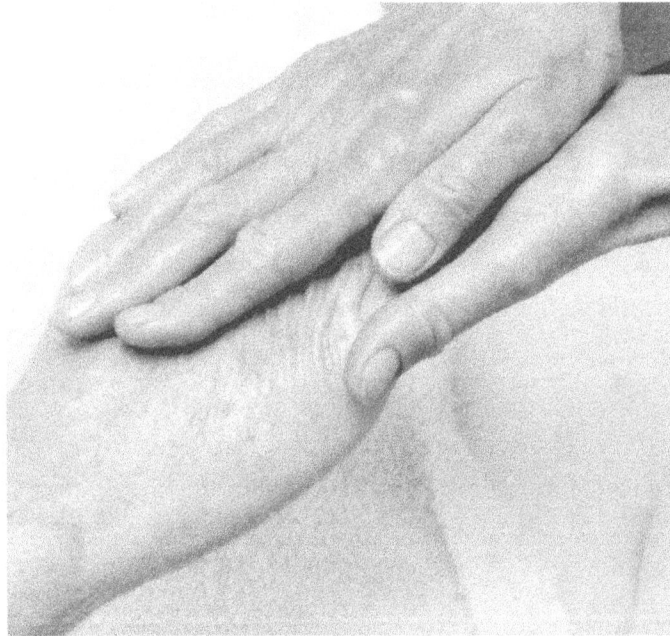

With hands over top of shoulder, effleurage the arm, gently flowing off fingertips

Now place your left hand on the left side of the 5th Thoracic Vertebra (about the top of the scapula region). Pull firmly through the Trapezius muscle, around the top of the Scapula (shoulder blade). Follow with your right hand.

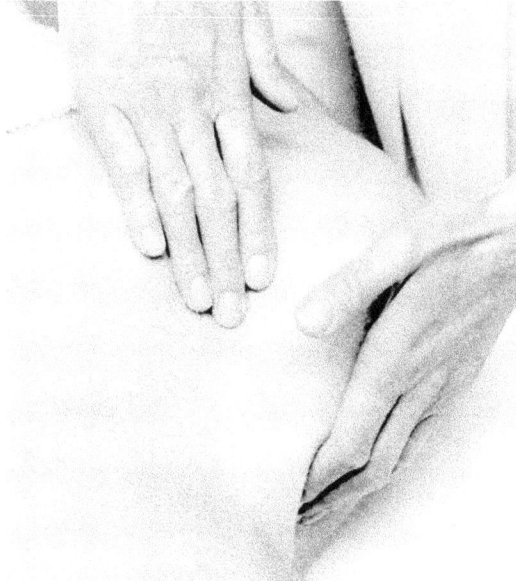

Pull firmly through the Trapezius then follow with the other hand

Petrissage the upper Trapezius, into the neck and out towards the shoulder. This petrissage takes determination to conquer due to the irregular positioning of muscles, your stance and both hands' movements. As you are still standing beside and facing the receiver, your right hand can petrissage quite easily however your left hand changes direction to move up the sides of the neck. Do not stand facing the receiver's feet as this makes the thumbs dig into the muscle. You need to apply this petrissage as you stand facing the receiver.

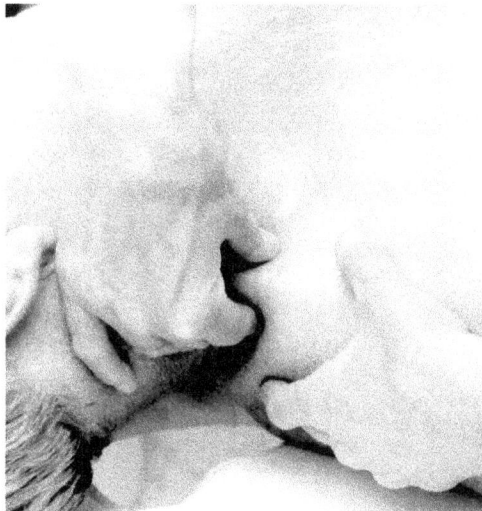

Petrissage the upper Trapezius

Separate the Deltoid by opening the thumb and index finger on your left hand to fit over the top of the shoulder. Glide down each side of the Deltoid muscle to the Deltoid insertion (about half way down the upper arm). You can feel where it ends. Now glide your right hand down and repeat, using both hands, one after the other.

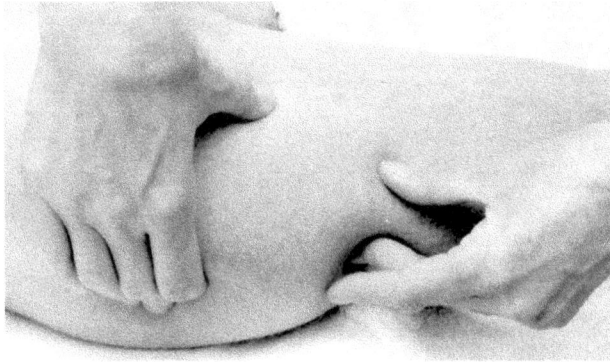

Separate the Deltoid. Glide down each side

Petrissage the Deltoid as you flow from separating straight into petrissage.

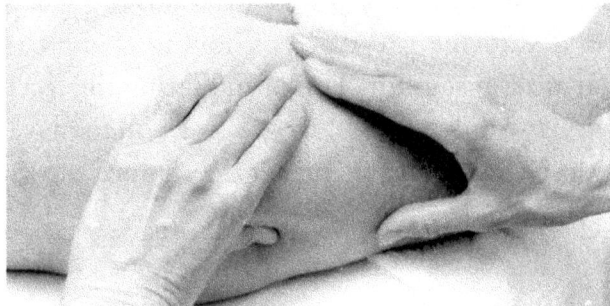

Petrissage the Deltoid

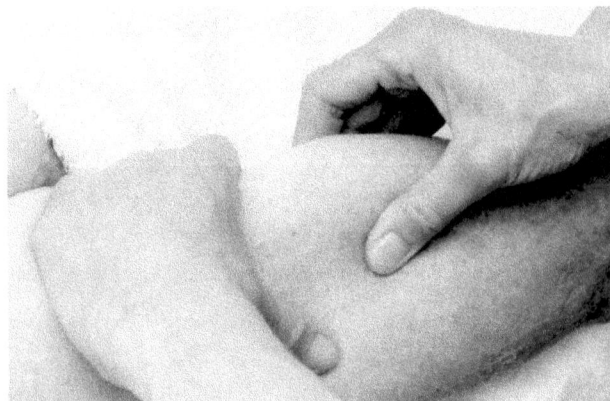

Petrissage the Biceps

Petrissage the Biceps, and then circle your left hand around the Head of the Humerus (bone at the top of the arm). Glide down under the arm to the elbow. Raise the receiver's elbow. Place it in your right hand and petrissage the Triceps with your left hand. Return the elbow and effleurage the arm and hand.

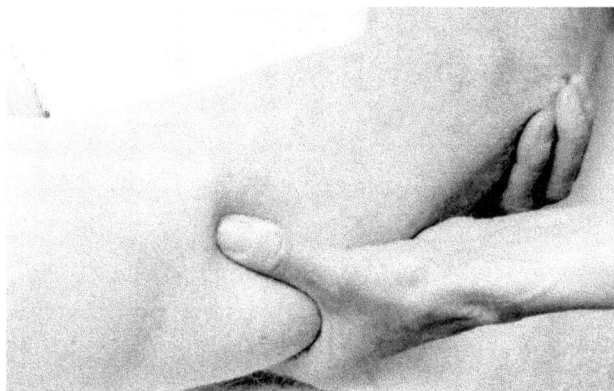

Petrissage the Triceps

LOWER ARM

Separate the Brachioradialis muscle from the Pronator Teres and Flexor Carpi Radialis. Using the indents on each side of the elbow as a guide, glide down the Brachioradialis. Maintain your rhythm. Petrissage the Brachioradialis.

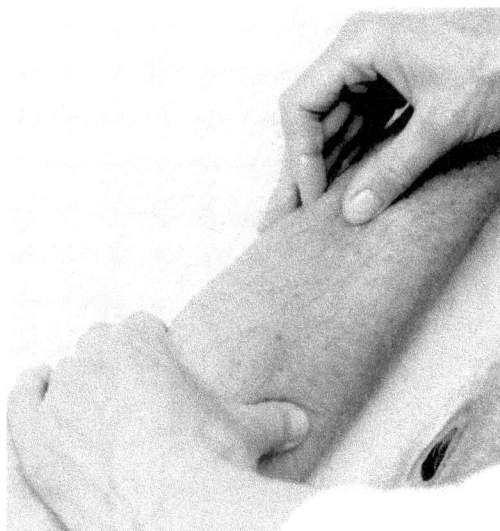

'Separate' the Brachioradialis

If the couch does not have an arm rest attached, sit on the edge of the couch, facing the receiver. If the arm is about to flop off the towel, lean sideways onto the edge of the couch and support the forearm as you separate and petrissage the Brachioradialis.

'Separate' the Radius and Ulna bones of the forearm. Place your left thumb at a right angle to the wrist. With right thumb following, glide up through the lower arm muscles to just below the elbow.

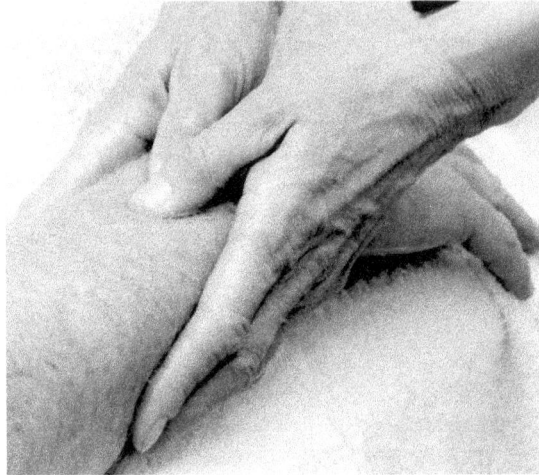

'Separate' the Radius and Ulna

Petrissage down the outer arm muscles as now your hands move one after the other from the elbow to the wrist.

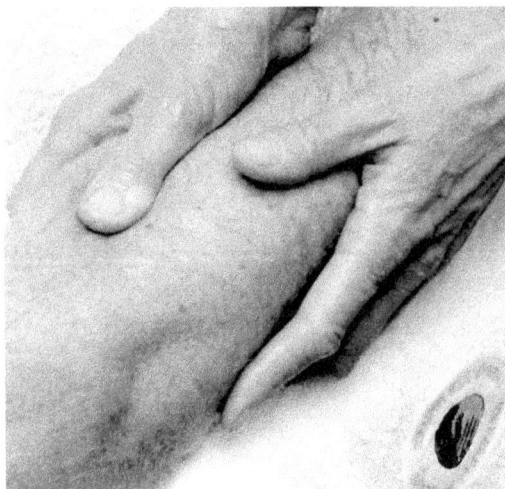

Petrissage the outer lower arm

Place a towel over your knees to avoid oil marking your garment or uniform. Rest the receiver's lower arm on the towel upon your thigh as you now work on the forearm. Your right knee is not under the same towel as the receiver's.

Place the palm of the receiver's hand to be facing upwards. Palpate the lower anterior forearm using the full flats of your thumbs, one after the other up along the Flexor Digitorum Superficialis, Flexor Carpi Ulnaris, Palmaris Longus, Flexor Carpi Radialis, Pronator Teres, Pronator Quadratus, Flexor Pollicis Longus and Abductor Pollicis Longus muscles.

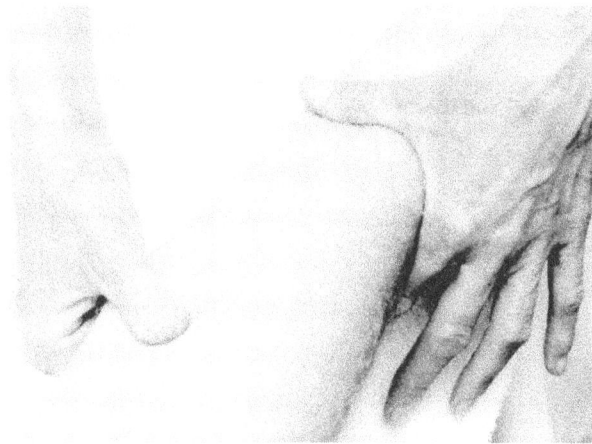

Palpate the inner forearm

Petrissage down the forearm to the wrist. Return the hand to the original resting position.

WRISTS AND HANDS

Effleurage the arm down to the wrists and palpate the Carpals (wrist) clockwise.

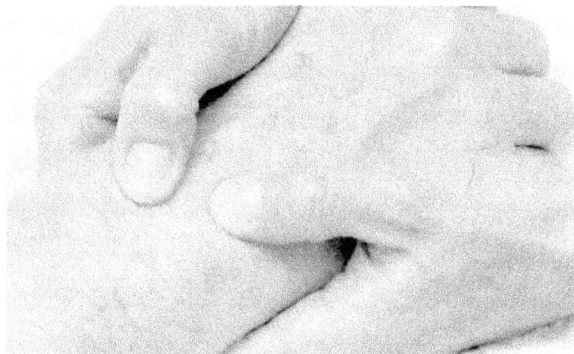

Palpate the Carpals

Metacarpals

Separate the Metacarpals (long bones between the wrist and fingers), remembering to apply all movements to the tolerance of the receiver. Take hold of the thumb and move it back and forth. Place your right thumb on the receiver's index finger and left thumb on the adjacent finger. With your fingers aligned on the palm, separate the Metacarpals. Move to the next finger and then the little finger.

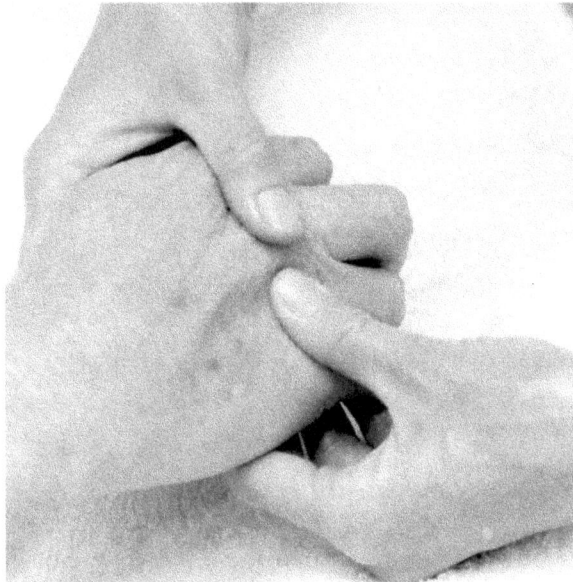

Separate the Metacarpals

Phalanges

Now standing facing the receiver's feet, squeeze each phalange (finger), one at a time, towards the palm. Place the ball of your right index finger onto the receiver's right thumb nail. Bend the first thumb joint as you are supporting and maintaining the largest knuckle straight with your left thumb and index finger. Squeeze towards the palm ensuring the large knuckle remains aligned with the metacarpal. Then straighten the phalange.

Move onto the index finger, squeezing it towards the palm. Follow along, bending each Phalange (finger), then straightening, including the little finger.

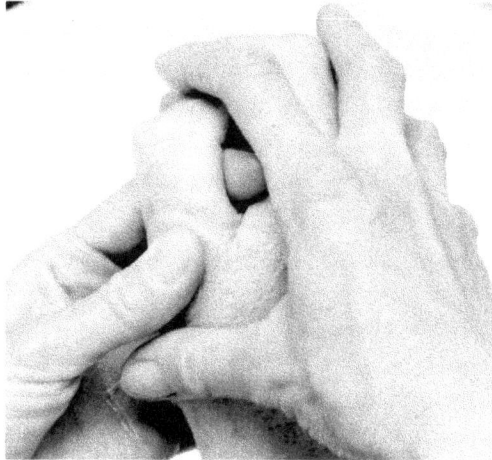

Place ball of index finger on thumb nail, supporting the largest knuckle

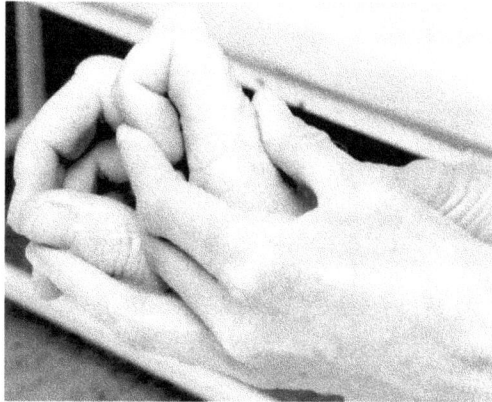

Squeeze towards the palm

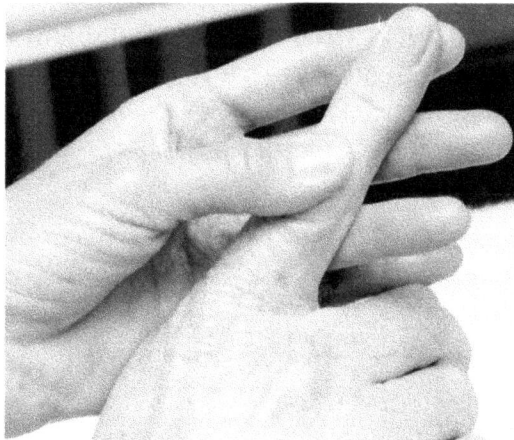

Straighten Phalange

Now place the tips of your fingers of your right hand on the receiver's right fingernails. Holding the large knuckles straight with the heel of your hand, squeeze fingertips simultaneously towards the receiver's palm until you feel resistance, hold for 5 seconds, and then release them.

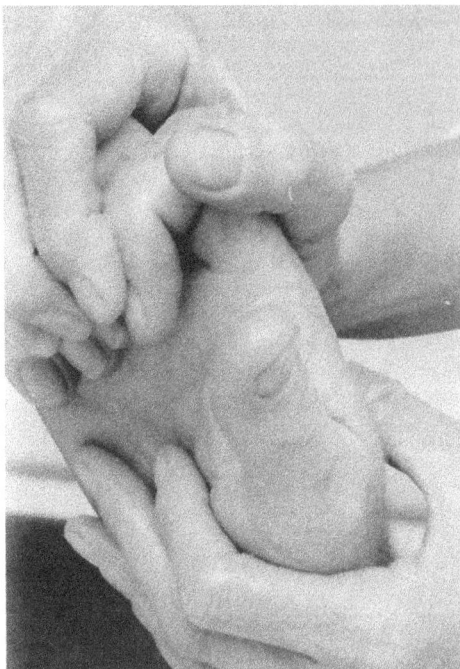

Squeeze fingers towards the palm

Carpals

Raise the receiver's hand. Supporting the forearm with your left hand, grasp the receiver's hand. Press upwards on the Metacarpal bones with your right hand and then press forward. Turn the hand side to side, and stretch the Carpals (wrist) at the same time.

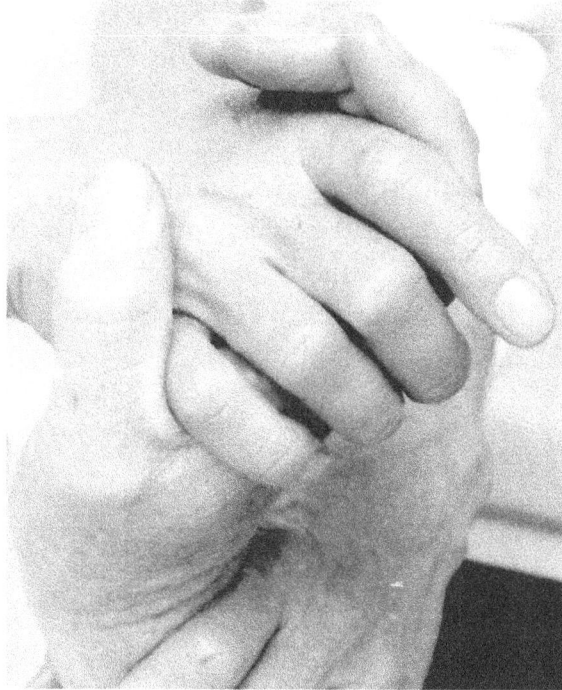

Press forward

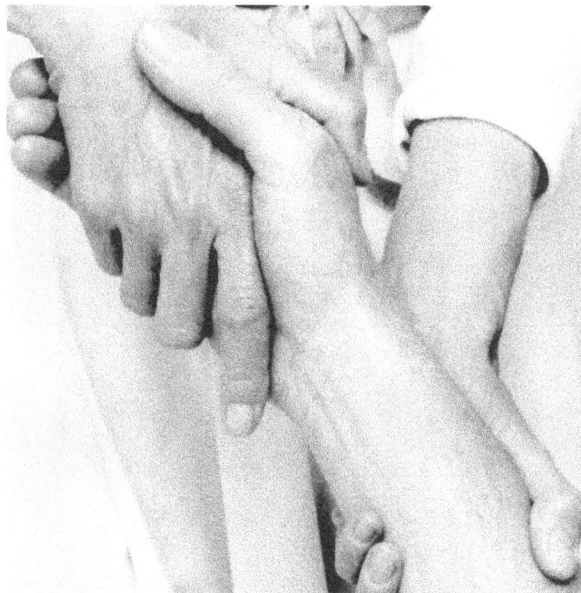

Turn hand side to side and stretch the Carpals

Rotate the wrist (Carpals). Grasp the hand and carefully turn it clockwise, then anti-clockwise. All of these joint moves aid in freeing any toxic residues that are or may be lying dormant.

Where there is a "breakout" at the joints or muscles, it usually means the area is overburdened with locked in toxins or foreign matter. Overuse of the surrounding muscles can also leave deposits of lactic acid creating pain. The circulation can be cut off from not wanting to do what the muscles have been applied to and as such, constant tension can be the cause of a 'breakout', usually created by a little voice in the subconscious mind saying, "I'm not good enough" that has come from an authority figure from the past. If this thought pattern isn't changed then arthritis can result. Additional healing methods are available in The Australian Advanced and Metaphysical Massage and Simple Foods to Heal Your Body. The receiver may feel instant relief to the area with these gentle moves.

Effleurage the hand. Rotate each Phalange (finger), stretching as you rotate. Repeat the hand effleurage. Finish with an effleurage of the arm and hand.

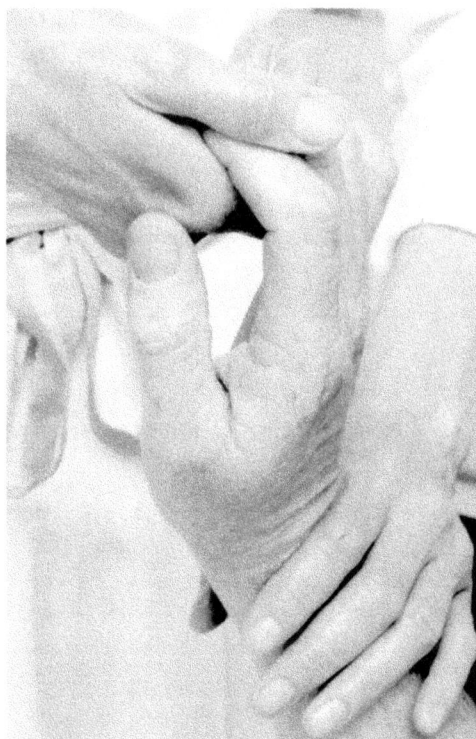

Stretch as you rotate each Phalange

Ensure to replenish fluids regularly with oxygenated, naturally alkaline and detoxified water. At least 8 glasses of filtered water or weak herbal teas (dependant on the climate) and physical exercise daily are necessary to move toxins through the body and out via the lymphatic and excretory systems.

If no swelling is evident, hot baths or compresses applied to stiff joints may also help heal the joints by way of bringing nutrition to these areas via the circulatory system.

SHOULDER ROTATION

Petrissage the Pectoralis Major (upper chest). Bring your fingers onto your palm (as in a fist shape) and petrissage by using the flats of both thumbs, one after the other.

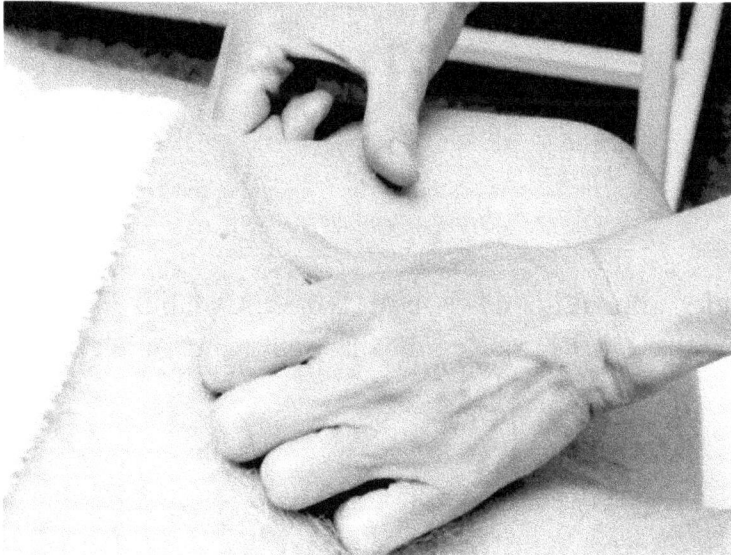

Petrissage the Pectoralis Major

Hold your hands as for chopping. Apply 2 splices (that's using the stiffened side of your little finger and hand) from the top of the Deltoid down across the Pectoralis Major to under the armpit.

Rotate the shoulder. Firstly, glide your left hand over the shoulder and down to the receiver's elbow. Supporting the elbow, bring the arm out and glide your right hand up to near the armpit. Hold the upper arm with your right hand. With your left hand now firmly on top of the shoulder, raise the arm with your right hand as you commence rotating clockwise. Press down on the shoulder with your left hand to complete the movement. Rotate the shoulder 3 times clockwise and 3 times anti-clockwise. This movement is used in remedial work and is described in more detail in The Australian Advanced and Metaphysical Massage.

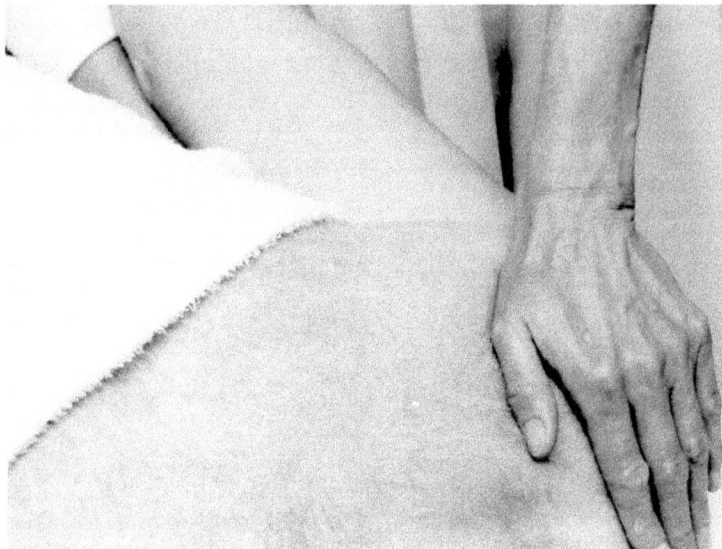

Rotate the shoulder

Effleurage the shoulder, arm and hand. Repeat Arms and Hands movements now on the left shoulder, arm and hand. Be sure to start with your right hand on left.

CHAPTER FOUR

FRONTS OF LEGS, ANKLES AND FEET

FRONT UPPER LEG

Arrange the towel for the front of the legs as per the back of the legs in Towel Tuck 2. Avoid all contact with the receiver's inner thigh.

If the room is warm you can apply oil to both legs. If it is cool, only apply oil to the leg you are about to work on and cover the other leg with another towel. Once again, check to see if the receiver is warm enough.

With right hand on left, commence effleurage on a 45° angle at mid-thigh. Effleurage the leg, applying firmer pressure up, lighter pressure down. Avoid the kneecap (Patella).

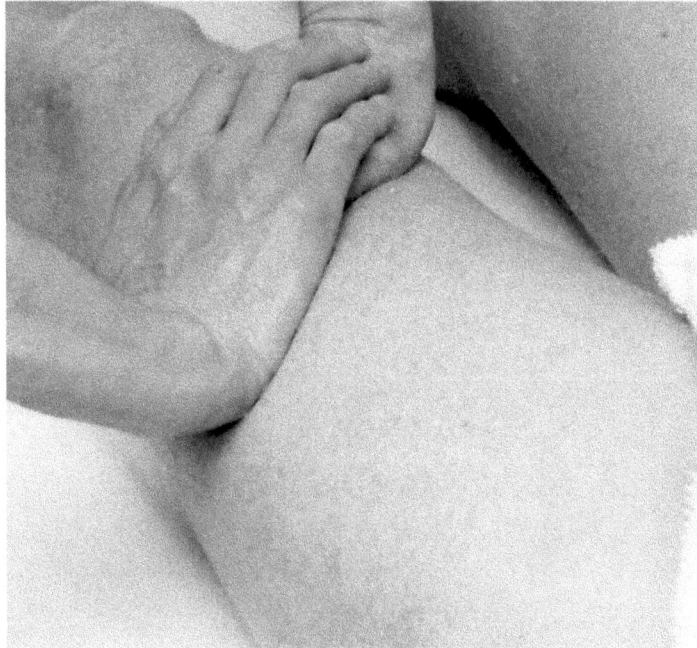

Effleurage the leg

Petrissage the Tensor Fasciae Latae muscle by bringing fingertips of your right hand up around the Neck of the Femur (between the Head of the Femur and the Greater Trochanter - similar to the back of the leg). Follow with your left fingertips. Repeat this move 3 times.

Petrissage the Quadriceps: Vastus Lateralis, Rectus Femoris, Sartorius, and Vastus Medialis muscles (thigh).

Cup the thigh, angling into the grains of the muscles (see quadriceps separation for muscle positions). To begin, face the receiver and bend your torso right over so that your head is at hand cupping level on the side of the receiver's leg. Move next to facing across the receiver's leg and continue cupping the middle, then upper inner knee.

Flick the thigh, following where you cupped the thigh muscles.

Effleurage the upper leg.

QUADRICEP SEPARATION

Separate the quadriceps (thigh). Bring your right index finger onto your palm and thumb is now the same height with a space of 2½ cm (1") between them. Place these two Phalanges at the indents above the receiver's left knee. Now glide up along the Rectus Femoris muscle to the top of the leg. Let the size of the muscle determine the distance between your thumb and index finger. Follow with your left hand.

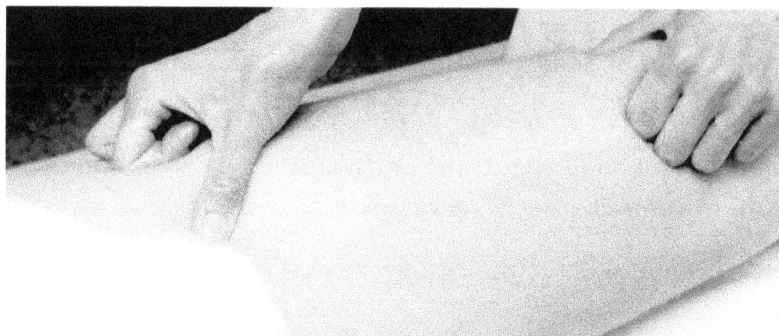

Glide up the Rectus Femoris (middle of thigh)

Retaining Phalange (thumb and index finger) position throughout the quadriceps separations, bring your right hand now to the outer side of the knee. Glide up along the Vastus Lateralis muscle. Now glide your left hand again up along the Rectus Femoris muscle. Follow with your right hand.

Place your left hand on the inner side of the knee and begin gliding up along the Sartorius muscle. Notice how it crosses over to the outside of the leg ¾ of the way up to the hip. This is the longest muscle in the body.

I found the easiest way for a student to remember these moves is by simply starting with the hand on the outside, then saying and following with "Middle, middle, outside, middle, middle, inside." Then repeat these movements.

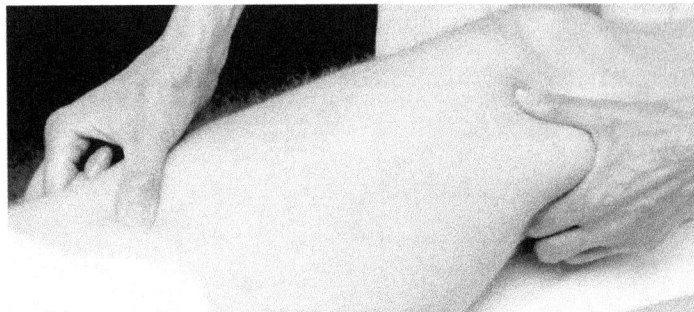

Glide up along the Sartorius
(commence at inner side of knee)

Effleurage the leg to the ankle (Tarsal bones).

FRONT LOWER LEG

Place your left thumb in front of your right thumb near the centre front of the lower leg, where the ankle bends on the left leg. Glide lightly up, beside the Tibia (shin bone), 'separating' it gently from the Tibialis Anterior muscle. Be aware of any varicose veins and surface veins present.

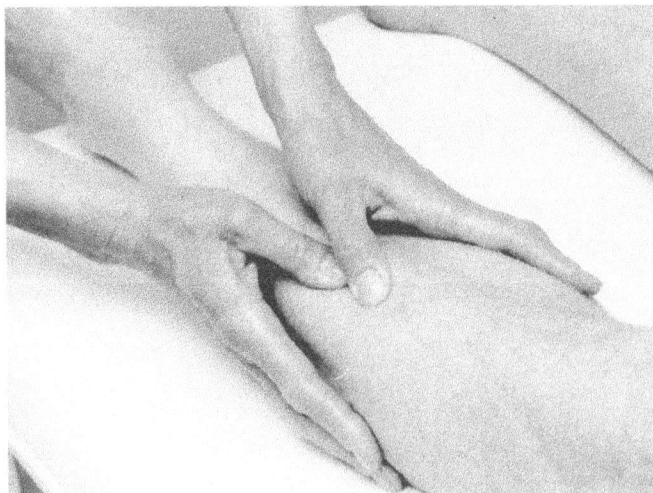

'Separate' the Tibialis Anterior

With your fingertips, glide gently up along the inner side of the Tibia (shin bone) separating it from the Soleus muscle.

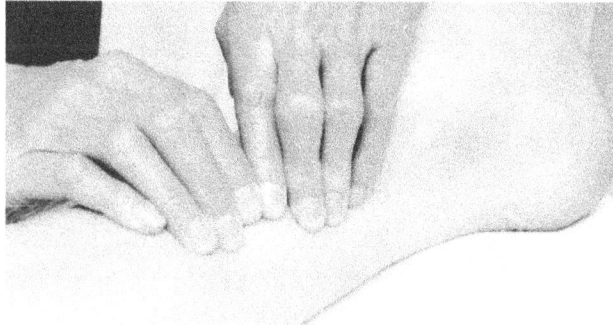

Glide along inner side of Tibia

Separate your hands just below the knee and petrissage down each side of the Tibia towards the ankle.

Raise the foot by placing your hand under the leg. Effleurage the lower leg. Glide hands in circles around both ankles (Tarsals), left hand anti-clockwise, right hand clockwise.

Now glide fingertips of your hand in and separate the side of the Tendon Calcaneus (large tendon between ankle and calf muscle). Changing hands, glide down and separate the other side of the Tendon Calcaneus using your fingertips.

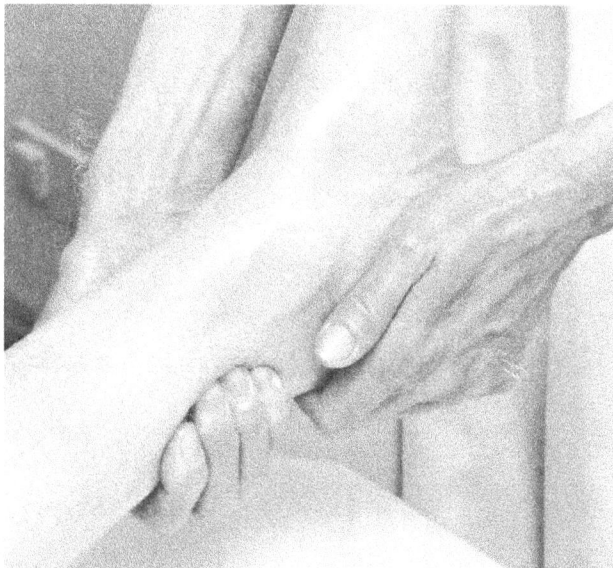

Separate the Tendon Calcaneus

Effleurage the lower leg. Apply a full leg effleurage down to the Tarsals (ankle bones) and roll directly into circular palpation of the ankle 3 times.

FRONT OF FOOT

Effleurage the foot. Facing the receiver's foot, separate the Metatarsals (long bones of the foot) and Phalanges (toes) by placing your thumbs on the largest knuckles of the big toe and adjacent toe. Your fingers are lined up behind, on the sole of the foot.

Press down with your right thumb and pull towards you with your left fingers. Now press down with your left thumb and pull towards you with your right fingers.

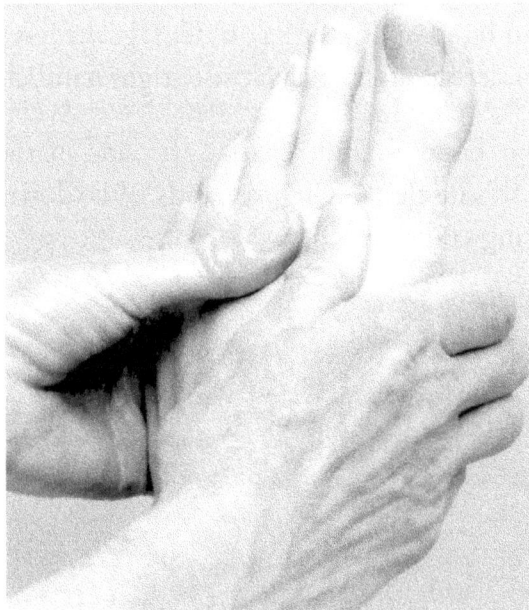

Separate the Metatarsals

Repeat both moves 3 times. Move along and separate the 2nd and 3rd Metatarsals (long bones of the foot); 3rd and 4th; 4th and 5th.

Glide between each Phalange (toe) with your thumbs. Lightly glide your left thumb across all of the large knuckles, commencing at the big toe joint across to the little toe.

JOINT STRETCHES

Stretch the Tendon Calcaneus (Achilles) by placing the heel of your hand on the ball of the foot. Your right hand supports the ankle. Now stretch the foot slowly forward, towards the leg, and then downwards, towards the couch. Remember to stretch only to the tolerance of the receiver. This stretch feels good on the Tendon Calcaneus and Tarsals and is a good move applied on athletes who enjoy the benefits of The Australian Massage the day prior to the big game, and is also beneficial after the big match.

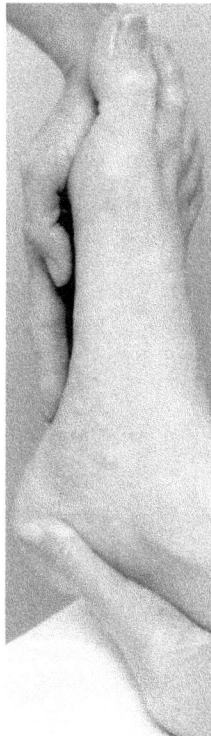

Stretch the Tendon Calcaneus

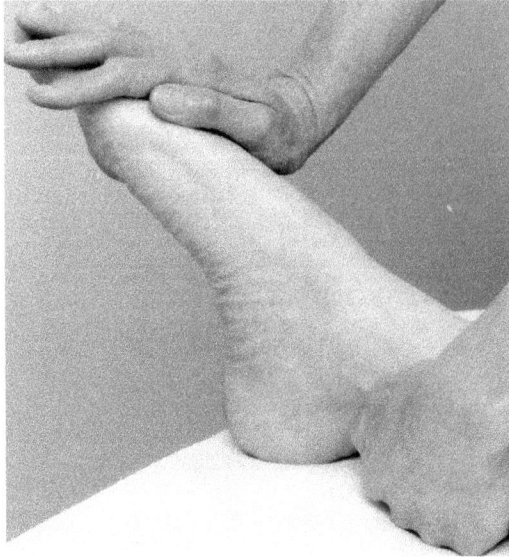

Stretch foot downwards

Rotate the Tarsals (ankle) by placing your right hand above the ankle and left hand around the centre of the foot. Turn the foot slowly clockwise, then anti-clockwise. Stretch all of the Phalanges (toes) at the same time by placing your thumb across all of the knuckles. Press the Phalanges (toes) forward, towards the couch. With your fingers, squeeze the Phalanges (toes) now towards the front of the leg.

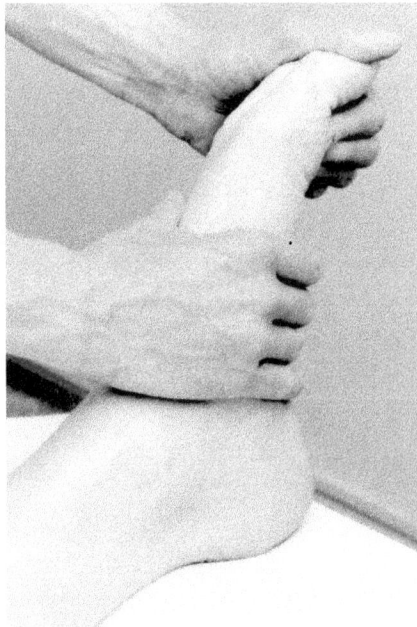

Stretch Phalanges forward

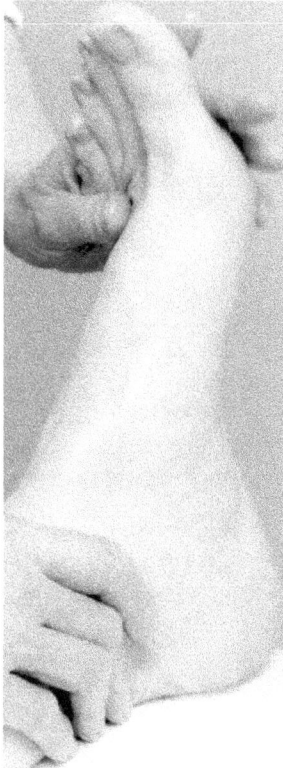

Squeeze Phalanges towards leg

Rotate and stretch the Phalanges. Grip the big toe. Rotate in a clockwise circular motion and stretch. Rotate and stretch the remaining Phalanges. Effleurage the leg and foot.

Change sides and repeat all of the leg and foot movements now on the receiver's right side. Remember to place your left hand on right to effleurage the right leg and foot, flowing serenely off the toes.

CHAPTER FIVE

NECK AND HEAD

NECK AND HEAD

FACE AND NECK PRE-CLEANSE

If the receiver has an excess of grime on the face or is wearing make-up, remove with a few drops of basic oil on cotton wads until a wad comes off the skin appearing to be clean.

Apply 10mL of basic oil which is suitable for facial skin, smoothing the oil upwards, to the front and back of the neck, upper Trapezius (between the back of the head and shoulder) and the face.

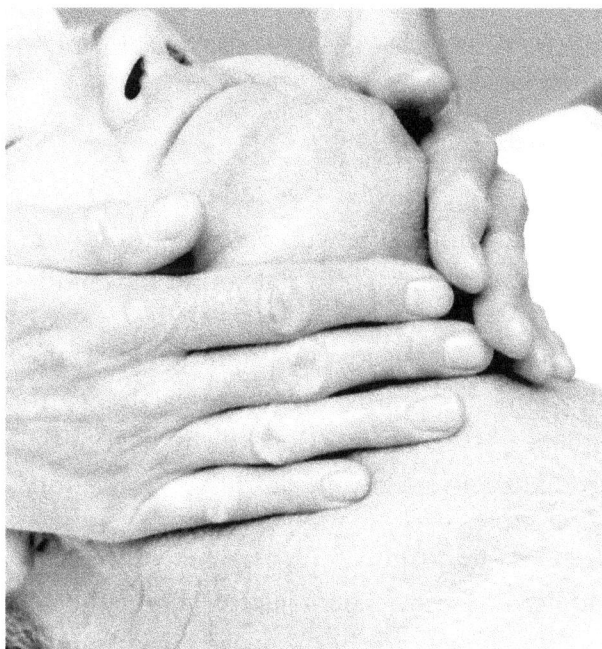

Smooth the oil upwards

NECK

Back of Neck

Effleurage the neck. Stand in front of the receiver's head facing the feet. Rest the head on your Rectus Abdominus muscle (lower abdomen) ensuring there are no buttons, clips or buckles to hinder the scalp. Check to see if the neck is relaxed. If the receiver is holding the head up, ask, "How much more are you able to relax your neck?" Using full palms, one in front of the other, effleurage the neck from the shoulder up to the hairline.

Palpate along each side of the Cervical Vertebrae. With right fingertips held firmly together, bring them onto the left side of the receiver's spine, down to as far you can reach, usually around the 2nd Thoracic Vertebra. This depends upon the length of your fingers or the receiver's neck. Your hands now fully support the head. Keeping fingernails well clear of the receiver's skin, glide up around each vertebra to the base of the skull. This move is one of the best for loosening the neck muscles. In The Australian Advanced and Metaphysical Massage you are shown how to apply specific stretches to the neck and direct palpation to free tightened muscles.

Change hands and repeat palpation along the right side of the Cervical Vertebrae with your left fingertips. Feel around each vertebra as you palpate along. Repeat palpation 3 times. Effleurage the neck and gently lower the head to the couch.

Front of Neck

Effleurage the front of the neck commencing with your right full palm on the right front side of the lowest point of the receiver's neck. Smoothly glide up to the chin just beneath the ear.

Now place your left full palm next to where your right palm commenced and glide up to the chin. Use these graceful neck effleurages working your way across, from one side of the neck to the other reaching to just beneath the receiver's left ear. Repeat neck effleurage commencing at the side where you finished, working your way back to where you first started.

Petrissage up the Sternocleidomastoid muscles in the front of the neck using one hand on each, commencing near the middle, just above the Clavicle. Avoid the hollow of the throat. Using thumbs and bent index fingers (similar to the quadriceps separation on the front of the thigh) petrissage up the more pronounced Sternocleidomastoid muscles. Follow these along to the base of the skull just behind the ears.

With hand held in this petrissage position, smoothly glide, in one move, commencing as for petrissage of the Sternocleidomastoid (above the Sternum or breastbone), right up to behind the ears.

FACE

Neck and Face Effleurage

Effleurage the neck and face. With left hand on right, place your right palm on the front of the lower neck. Effleurage up the neck to the chin. Commence separating both hands as you also separate index fingers and adjacent fingers to let the receiver's chin slide between them into the diamond shaped opening. Continue the effleurage over both sides of the face up to the forehead.

With fingers together, place the heel of both hands on each side of the receiver's forehead above the eyes. Now glide with an upward outward sweep to the Temporalis muscle (temple) and gently float off the forehead.

Petrissage the face using the sides of and balls of both thumbs and first two fingers. Commence petrissage at the centre forehead. Moving clockwise, petrissage down the left side of the face, around the chin, then petrissage up along the right side of the face to the centre forehead where you first started.

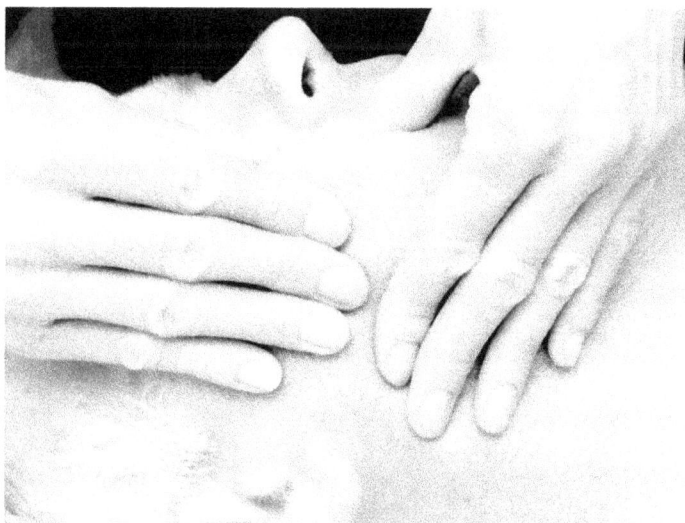

Petrissage the face

Sinus Palpation

Palpate the sinuses. Hold the balls of your thumbs on the Frontal Sinuses region at the centre of the forehead, between the eyes and above the nose, for 3 seconds and release. Raise thumbs and place them on the Ethmoid Sinus region at the sides of the top of the nose. Be aware of the nasal passages and allow air to circulate freely. Ensure they remain open at all times. Hold for 3 seconds and release. Glide downwards, palpating the Maxillary Sinuses around the Zygomatic bones (cheeks) extending out to the ears, following around the cheek bones.

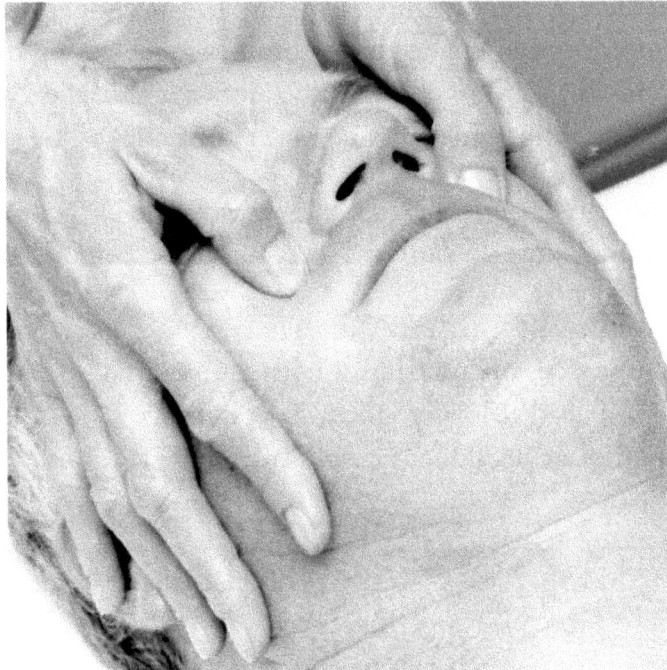

Palpate the Sinuses

In the event of nasal blockages caused by mucus, a film that gathers around foreign matter, give a cup of peppermint green tea after The Australian Massage. Never apply peppermint, eucalyptus or tea tree oils of any type to the facial skin around the eyes as either can cause inflammation to the eyes.

Glide thumbs, one after the other up along the nose and lightly across the tip of nose.

Effleurage the neck and face in one complete uplifting movement.

Palpate the Temporalis muscle on each side of the forehead. Place the balls of your first 3 fingers of both hands on the Temporalis muscles. Palpate left hand clockwise, right hand anti-clockwise. Avoid gliding across the receiver's skin.

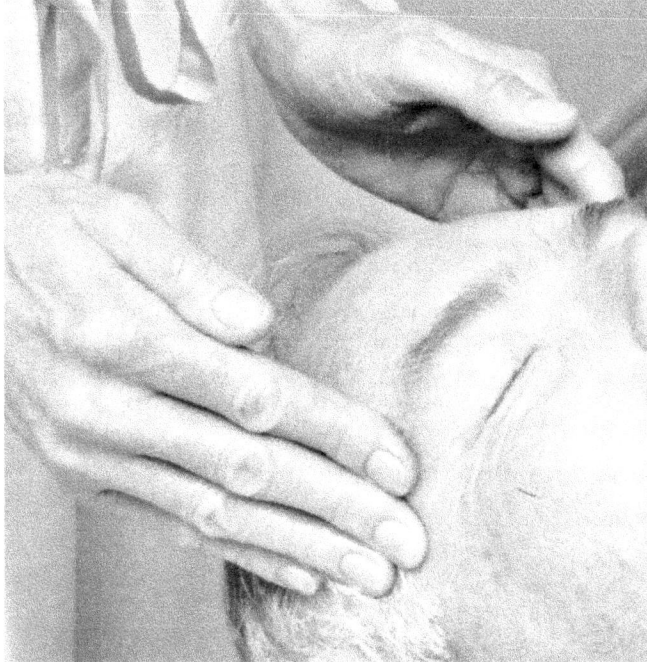

Palpate the Temporalis (temples)

Smooth over closed eyes. Using thumbs, smooth across the receiver's closed eyes, commencing near the nose. Glide across the eyes, following the contours if the eyelashes, up to the outer corner of the eye brows.

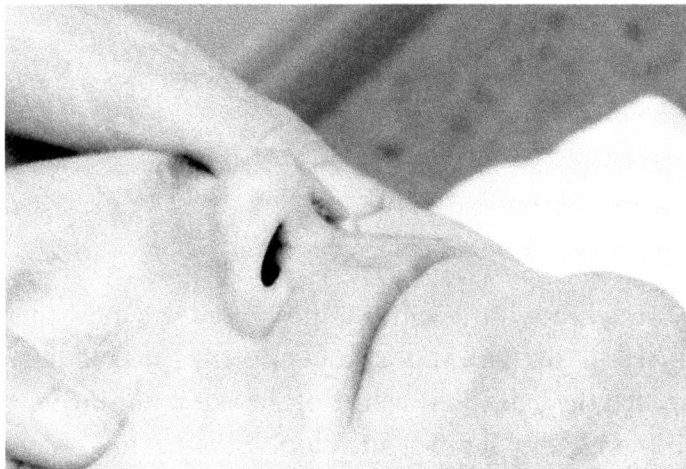

Smooth over closed eyes

Effleurage the neck and face.

SCALP

Scalp Effleurage

Ask the receiver if it is fine to have oil in the hair. If the answer is, "No," wash your hands thoroughly and dry at this point in time.

Effleurage the scalp. Separate your first two fingers from your thumbs, holding the last three fingers pressed together. Place your opened fingers with the receiver's ears between them. Now place your thumbs at the centre forehead. Spread remaining fingers widely apart.

Firmly draw your fingers and thumbs through the hair to the centre of the scalp without pulling out any of the receiver's hair.

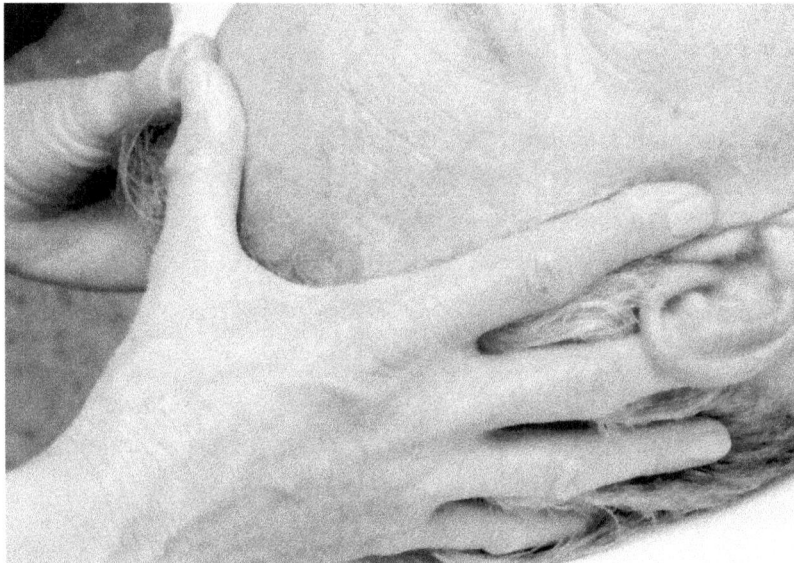

Effleurage the scalp

To easily raise the receiver's head, lift it with the heel of your hands, then place spread fingers around the back of the head. Now with your spread fingertips around the base of the skull bone, Effleurage upwards through the hair to the centre of the skull, uniting with the thumbs. Placing one of your feet on the lower bar under the couch top (if there is one) is most useful for applying head and some neck moves.

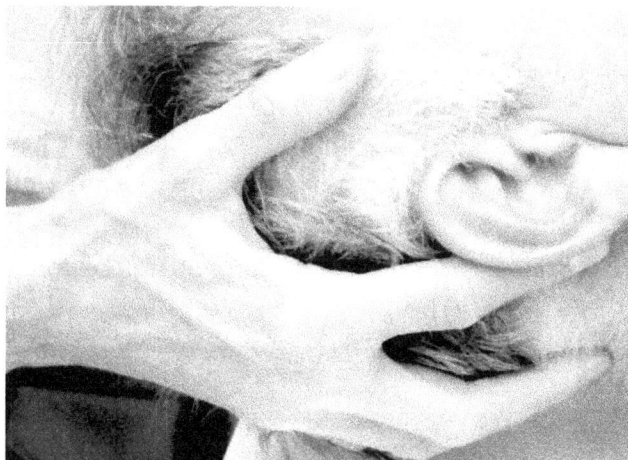

Effleurage from base of skull

Scalp Palpation

Palpate the scalp. Hold your hands in the same position as for the first scalp effleurage. Palpate with fingertips, using your thumb for guidance. Apply with small, circular, firm palpation movements: right hand clockwise, left hand anti-clockwise. Follow the same path as for the scalp effleurage to the centre of the scalp, palpating all the way. Now palpate from the base of the scalp up to the centre.

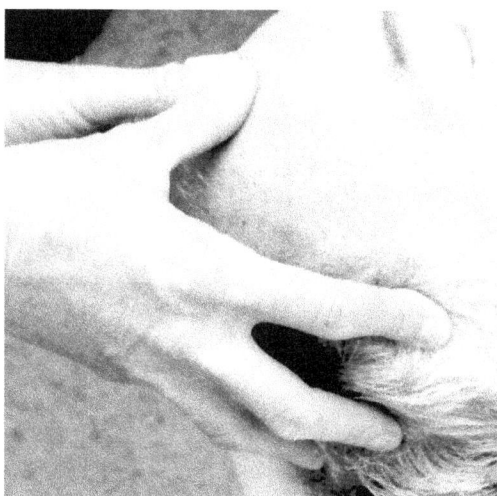

Palpate with fingertips

Palpate the centre of the scalp. Standing now beside and facing the receiver's head, glide your fingers between each other allowing the fingertips to rest where the palm begins. Now place thumbs side by side on the central forehead. With fingertips slightly separated on the centre scalp, palpate the area. Follow with a full scalp effleurage.

Palpate the exterior of the muscle motor area of the brain. Feel for the delicate indent situated slightly in front of the centre scalp. Without gliding across the skin and hair, calmly and very slowly palpate clockwise with your little finger.

This has a powerful impact on the central nervous system and muscle co-ordination after The Australian Massage. Gradually lighten your touch as you palpate. Become lighter, lighter, lighter, and lighter – until there is no physical contact at all. Performed as I have instructed and shown, at this point the receiver isn't even aware that you have finished, simply floating in their world of bliss, yet down to earth and ready to move forward lovingly into their own wonderful world.

THE COMPLETION

The receiver feels so relaxed now and knows what Heaven feels like on Earth. Let the receiver know you are leaving the room for a short time and for her/him to relax until you return. Quietly leave the room for a few minutes and allow the receiver to relish in the blissful floating sensation (and the delicate, delightful aroma if you used a few drops of an essential oil with the basic oil). If the couch is portable, do not leave the room, and now gently assist the receiver in sitting upright (see next paragraph). Support a lightweight framed portable couch so that it does not tip over.

If upon your return, the receiver has fallen asleep, gently awaken by saying, "…….. (Name), can you hear me? You can rise from the couch now." Stay and support the receiver to sitting-up position on the side of the couch. Say, "I'm going to assist you in sitting up now."

Standing on the left side of the couch place your right hand under the back of the receiver's neck and the right arm over the top of the receiver's right knee and place your hand under the right knee. Gently slide the receiver's legs from the knees down over the edge of the couch as you assist in the sitting up process.

The receiver may feel light-headed or giddy when first sitting up. This can occur if you applied The Australian Massage too swiftly. If you see the face is white stand behind the receiver. Gently lower the head forward. Effleurage up the neck to replenish blood supply to the head.

If the face is red, effleurage down the neck and drain away excess blood from the head towards the heart. Always remain with the receiver until the head is clear.

Sometimes the eyes may appear puffy. This means the body requires balance. To achieve this, diet and activities need to be adjusted accordingly. Ask the receiver to repeat this affirmation, "I have a healthy, balanced body," and to allow the intelligence within the body to take care of the rest.

While the receiver is showering and/or dressing, clean your work area. If there is any unused massage oil remaining, absorb this in a paper towel and drop into the bin. Wherever you store discarded oiled paper or cloths ensure it is in a cool area as some oils are flammable when heated.

It is advisable not to re-use preheated massage oil. After a few massages you will become familiar with the correct quantity required per person.

Give the receiver a drink of ultra-finely filtered water.

Upon completion, always wash your hands and clean your fingernails with antiseptic wash such as tea tree soap and drink a glass or two of finely filtered water to replenish your fluids. The human body contains around 70% water so make sure you replenish fluids with Mother Nature's best.

Paradise Waters Pty Ltd produces RAINFOREST DEW™, Australia's original bottled rainwater manufactured for commercial use and is totally compatible with the blood stream. It has qualities that differ to all other types of water. The factory, established in October 1995, is located amidst the pristine rainforest region of the wet tropics at Japoonvale, in North Queensland.

More information is available on the topic of water in my book Simple Foods to Heal Your Body.

This completes The Australian Massage and thank you for joining me.

The Magic In Touch Is Beautiful

And So Are You

Always Love Your Body
And Your Body Will Respond With Vibrant Energy

About Chapter Six and The Australian Massage Video, DVD or Cassette

Chapter Six is designed to make learning so much easier. By having these simplified movements on a reading stand close to your working couch, bench or table, learning is simplified for beginner students, and even more so if you have The Australian Massage Therapy Video or DVD to watch or the Cassette to listen to.

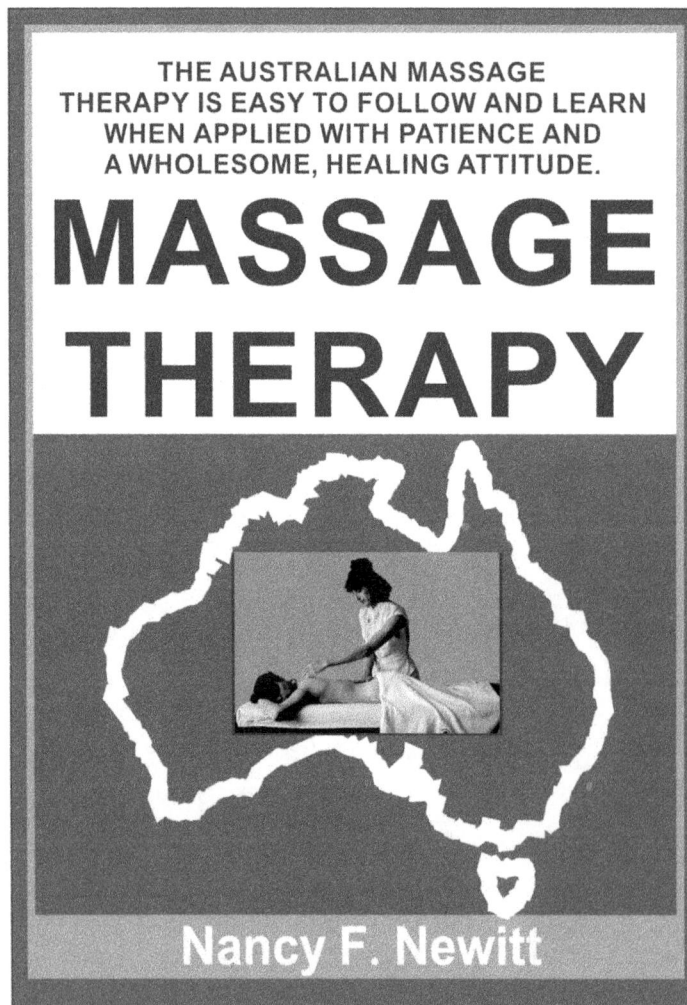

THE AUSTRALIAN MASSAGE THERAPY IS EASY TO FOLLOW AND LEARN WHEN APPLIED WITH PATIENCE AND A WHOLESOME, HEALING ATTITUDE.

MASSAGE THERAPY

Nancy F. Newitt

CHAPTER SIX

QUICK TIPS

MOVEMENTS OF THE BACK

1. Oil the Back

2. Effleurage the Back

3. Petrissage the Trapezius

4. Palpate the Neck

5. Palpate the Base of the Skull

6. Effleurage the Back

7. Palpate the Shoulder muscles and Deltiod

8. Cup and Flick the Shoulder and Deltoid

9. Smooth over and Separate the Scapula from Ribs

10. Repeat 8 and 9 on the other side

11. Effleurage the Back

12. Palpate between Spine and Longitudinal Muscles

13. Roll across the Longitudinal Muscles

14. Roll Full Palms across the Back

15. Effleurage the Back

16. Separate the Ribs

17. Figure 8 of the Back and Deltoids

18. Effleurage the Back

19. Finish lightly over the Deltoids

MOVEMENTS OF THE LEGS (BACK)

1. Oil the Legs

2. Effleurage the Leg

3. Petrissage the Upper Leg

4. Cup and Flick the Upper Leg

5. Effleurage the Upper Leg

6. Effleurage the Leg

7. Petrissage the Lower Leg

8. Cup and Flick the Lower Leg

9. Effleurage the Lower Leg

10. Effleurage the Leg

11. Separate the Gastrocnemius muscle (calf)

12. Effleurage the Leg and Foot

13. Separate the Achilles Tendon and Soleus muscle (above ankle)

14. Effleurage and Palpate the Tarsals ((ankle bones)

15. Effleurage the Foot

16. Figure 8 on the Sole of the Foot

17. Flick the Sole

18. Effleurage the Sole

19. Separate the Metatarsals (between ankle and toes)

20. Roll thumb across the large knuckles

21. Effleurage the Foot

22. Effleurage the Leg and Foot

23. Repeat movements 1 to 21 on the other leg and foot

24. Figure 8 of the Back and Deltoids

25. Effleurage the Back

26. Finish gently off the Deltoids

MOVEMENTS OF THE ARMS AND HANDS

1. Oil the Upper Trapezius (top of upper back and neck) and Arms

2. Effleurage the Arm and Hand

3. Petrissage the Trapezius

4. Separate and Petrissage the Deltoid

5. Petrissage the Biceps (front of upper arm)

6. Petrissage the Triceps (back of upper arm)

7. Separate and Petrissage the Brachioradialis (front of forearm below the elbow)

8. Separate the Radius and Ulna (lower arm bones) then Petrissage

9. Palpate and Petrissage the Inner Forearm

10. Palpate the Carpals (wrist)

11. Separate the Metacarpals (long bones of the palm)

12. Squeeze Phalanges (fingers) towards the Palm

13. Stretch and Rotate the Carpals

14. Stretch and Rotate the Phalanges

15. Effleurage the Arm and Hand

16. Petrissage the Pectoralis Major

17. Rotate the Shoulder

18. Effleurage the Arm

19. Repeat Movements 1 to 18 on the other Arm

MOVEMENTS OF THE LEGS (FRONT)

1. Oil the Legs

2. Effleurage the Leg

3. Petrissage the Upper Leg

4. Cup and Flick the Upper Leg

5. Effleurage the Upper Leg

6. Effleurage the Leg

7. Separate the Quadriceps (Front upper leg muscles)

8. Effleurage the Leg

9. Separate and Petrissage each side of the Tibia (shin)

10. Effleurage and Palpate the Lower Leg

11. Effleurage the Leg and Palpate the Tarsals (ankle bones)

12. Effleurage the Foot

13. Separate the Metatarsals and Phalanges (toes)

14. Stretch the Phalanges

15. Stretch the Foot

16. Rotate the Tarsals

17. Stretch and Rotate the Phalanges

18. Effleurage the Leg and Foot

19. Repeat Movements 1 to 18 on the other Leg

MOVEMENTS OF THE NECK AND HEAD

1. Effleurage the Back of the Neck

2. Palpate the Cervical Vertebrae (back of the neck)

3. Effleurage the Neck

4. Effleurage the Front of the Neck

5. Petrissage the Sternocleidomastoid (long muscle from breastbone to behind ears)

6. Effleurage the Neck and Face

7. Petrissage the Face muscles

8. Palpate the Sinuses

9. Palpate the Nose

10. Effleurage the Neck and Face

11. Palpate the Temporalis (temples)

12. Smoothly glide over closed Eyes

13. Effleurage the Neck and Face

14. Effleurage the Scalp

15. Palpate the Scalp

16. Effleurage the Scalp

17. Finish with Palpation at Centre of Scalp

IN-DEPTH BODY INFORMATION

Corresponding Areas of the Body Connected to Nerves from the Spinal Chord

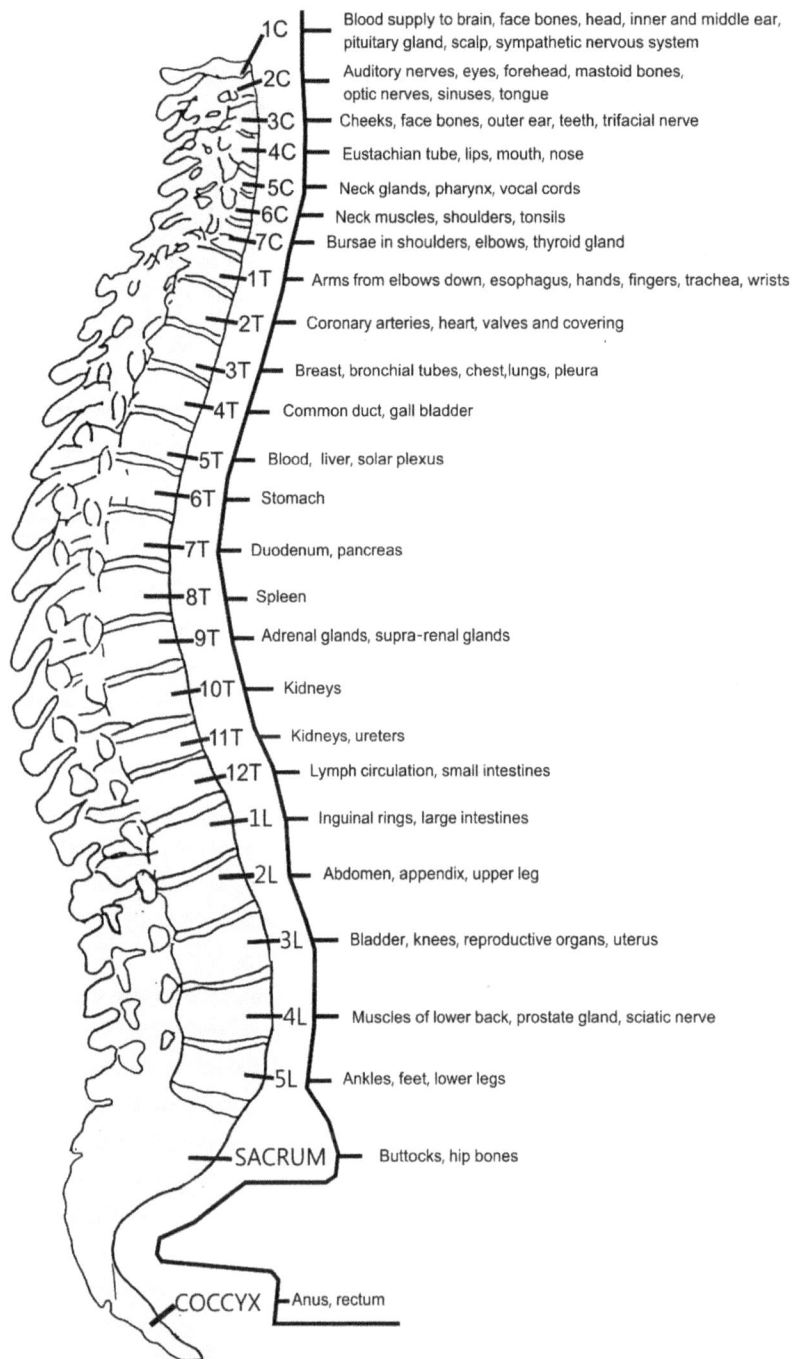

Vertebra	Corresponding Area
1C	Blood supply to brain, face bones, head, inner and middle ear, pituitary gland, scalp, sympathetic nervous system
2C	Auditory nerves, eyes, forehead, mastoid bones, optic nerves, sinuses, tongue
3C	Cheeks, face bones, outer ear, teeth, trifacial nerve
4C	Eustachian tube, lips, mouth, nose
5C	Neck glands, pharynx, vocal cords
6C	Neck muscles, shoulders, tonsils
7C	Bursae in shoulders, elbows, thyroid gland
1T	Arms from elbows down, esophagus, hands, fingers, trachea, wrists
2T	Coronary arteries, heart, valves and covering
3T	Breast, bronchial tubes, chest, lungs, pleura
4T	Common duct, gall bladder
5T	Blood, liver, solar plexus
6T	Stomach
7T	Duodenum, pancreas
8T	Spleen
9T	Adrenal glands, supra-renal glands
10T	Kidneys
11T	Kidneys, ureters
12T	Lymph circulation, small intestines
1L	Inguinal rings, large intestines
2L	Abdomen, appendix, upper leg
3L	Bladder, knees, reproductive organs, uterus
4L	Muscles of lower back, prostate gland, sciatic nerve
5L	Ankles, feet, lower legs
SACRUM	Buttocks, hip bones
COCCYX	Anus, rectum

LATERAL VIEW

Spinal vertebrae that are out of alignment may cause irritation to the nervous system.

Relaxation created by The Australian Massage changes the affects that mis-alignments have on the structure, organs and bodily functions therefore assisting in natural re-alignment of spinal vertebrae.

CHAPTER SEVEN

THE AROMAS OF NATURE
ESSENTIAL OIL FAMILIES
PURE AND NATURAL
HERBS AND APPLICATIONS

THE AROMAS OF NATURE

Essential Oil Families

Plants belong to families and becoming familiar with what you may use occasionally gives a closer understanding of what they are. This chapter provides only a very small glimpse into herbal oils. There are good references in "Useful Websites" that you may like to research and extend your knowledge on oils. Always be on the lookout for 100% pure and natural essential oils to use.

GRAMINAE (earth)

Graminae family members e.g. citronella, lemongrass, litsea cubeba, palmarosa and vetiver; show an astonishing adaptability, resilience and flexibility. The ability to cover large areas indicates its outstanding strength which is located in the powerful root system, forming a complex network.

The Graminae is governed by long narrow leaves and straight stems. This family disburses little energy in the flowering process. This nutritious family with its leaves and seeds provide to the animals e.g. grass for herbivorous animals, grains for humans, birds, rats and mice.

Vetiver produces essential oil in its roots whereas the other herbs with their fresh, green, lemony and slightly rosy fragrance produce there oils in the stems, leaves and seeds.

CONIFERAE (air – light, inner warmth verses cold)

Coniferae family members e.g. cedarwood, cypress, fir, juniper, pine and spruce thuja; are best at home in the frigid and temperate zones of the north and south hemispheres. They only grow best at high altitudes in tropical regions.

The obviousness of this family is dominated by a vertical and linear principle. Everything is structured around the vertical trunk which is surrounded with branches like little trees themselves and leaves that reduce to long needles. These needles are in spirals around twigs. A cone of flowers is reduced to its minimum of a terminal twig surrounded by dense leaves resembling wood. It also bears the stamens or pistil on the leaves' axil.

The oldest and highest trees in the world belong to the Coniferae family. Their timber (e.g. cypress) was once used to make furniture. In some species, the trunks are virtually immune to rot. Their etheric oils and resins are produced in abundance. In some species resin production is so intense that the trees exude it through their trunks or cones, indicating a deep relationship with the forces of warmth and light.

COMPOSITAE (light)

Compositae family members are identified by a collection of petite flowers that form an incomparable superior entity. With its simple and basic structure, Compositae constitutes the largest botanical family. Another large family with brilliant floral variations are orchids. Compositae, being intensely related to light, live primarily in the floral sphere. The plants therapeutic action shows immense diversity. Compositae grow all over the world.

BURSERACEAE (dry fire)

Burseraceae family members grow in desert tropical areas e.g. elemi, frankincense and myrrh. They draw on the intense cosmic activity that stimulates the formation of gum and etheric oils. Growing in the most extreme climate on the planet are myrrh and frankincense. Burseraceae condense the energy of the desert. A thin layer of essential oil filters the sun's rays while it freshening the air around them. They have strong anti-inflammatory actions. Putrefaction cannot take place because the air is too dry and the fire too intense. They have powerful healing properties when there is intense burning in the body, acting against it. Acting against burning it is used especially for controlling secretions. They also have a strong effect on corpses, a beneficial action on ulcers, gangrene, gastric, and intestinal fermentation.

LABIATAE (heat)

Labiatae family members influence the universal forces of heat e.g. basil, clary sage, hyssop, lavender, lavandin, marjoram, Melissa, oregano, patchouli, pennyroyal, peppermint, rosemary, sage, spearmint, spike and thyme. Labiatae prefer median climatic areas and love open spaces such as dry, rocky slopes and sunny hills or mountains. Because of their affinity for the digestive processes, these culinary herbs are invigorating, stimulating, fiery and reawakening with natural fragrances.

MYRTACEAE (fire, air, water, earth – harmony)

Myrtaceae family members grow in the tropics where they are confronted with the powerful forces of earth and water in relation to strong tropical domination. Myrtaceae does not produce any poisonous plant therefore has a noble and harmonious aspect, expressing the perfect equilibrium among the four elements; water, fire, earth and air. Strong and simple evergreen leaves open themselves to the supra vegetal and animal sphere in an intense floral process.

Myrtaceae examples are bay, cajeput, clove, eucalyptus, myrtle, niaouli, nutmeg, tea tree and red pepper, with fruits such as gooseberry, guava, myrtoloela fruits, jabotica plums and pomegranate. Deeply penetrated into the leaf, flower, bark and wood, generating etheric oils and aromatic resins is the tropical warmth. Revealing its healthy relation with the earth, Myrtaceae produces very hard woods.

RUTACEAE (subdued heat)

Rutaceae family members generally grow in the tropics e.g. bergamot, grapefruit, lemon, lime, orange, petitgrain, tangerine and rue (highly toxic). With hard wood that is often resinous and with green firm leaves, Rutaceae are mostly small thorny trees. The fragrance exhaled from their beautiful abundant star-shaped flowers is delicious, exhilarating and sweet. The leaves provide a fresh scent that is comforting with a hint of bitterness. Rutaceae, activated by air and warmth, produce juicy, acid fruits or small hot, spicy berries.

UMBELLIFERAE (air)

Umbelliferae family members are characterised by the extreme division of the leaves which end up in an aerial alikeness e.g. anise and fennel. Other members consist of angelica, aniseed, caraway, carrot, coriander, cumin, lovage, celery and parsley. Umbelliferae gives birth to a strong root system which stays underground for one or more years by using the interaction of air, light, water and earth through exceedingly developed leaves. Umbelliferae's fructification process begins in the leaves and root to produce tasty vegetables and condiments. Umbelliferae have an affinity for the digestive system, a strong action on the glandular system and secretions.

PURE AND NATURAL

The best guarantee of quality is to obtain essential from a specialist supplier who has an in-depth knowledge of essential oils and their production techniques.

All essential oils can be stored in the dark at a reasonable ambient temperature. Storage in the refrigerator is not recommended as this may cause specific chemicals to solidify and precipitate thereby rendering the remaining oil less complete (e.g. citrus bergamia). Some oils (e.g. pimpinella anisum) will freeze at relatively high temperatures. In this event, the oil must be gently heated until it is fully liquid and well shaken before being used.

Genuine and authentic essential oils must be derived from plants of specific species. Reference is made to the fact that "Genuine and Authentic" oils come from plants that are produced by superior growing and distillation techniques. These are the techniques used in the production of true "100% Pure and Natural" oils.

Genuine and authentic oils are produced by slow distillation processes and preferably at reduced pressure. This is implicit in a guarantee of pure and natural in its true sense and is achieved by dealing only with the best and most reputable producers in the world today and the choice of oils for their quality.

Three commonly used essential oils blends known as Ylang Ylang, Patchouli and Sandalwood are often adulterated.

Many oils are adulterated with turpentine which itself is adulterated with petroleum, rosin spirit and volatile portions of shale oil and coal tar.

Price is often a reasonable guideline when buying essential oils. Beware of oils that are cheap. This does not necessarily mean that the oil must be expensive to be good. Genuine and authentic essential oils must not be decolourised, recoloured or deterpenated (refer to Useful Websites Ahimsa).

HERBS AND APPLICATIONS

Basic Herbal Preparations

INFUSION

To make an infusion, place 1½ handfuls of fresh herbs or 25gms (1oz) of dried herb into a saucepan (not aluminium or copper). Bring 570mL (1 pint) of filtered rainwater to the boil. Pour over the herb and cover with a lid, preventing the loss of any volatile elements through evaporation. Simmer for 30 minutes. Strain and store in the refrigerator for up to 3 days.

DECOCTION

Decocting is the best method for tougher roots, barks, stems or seeds. Place 25gms (1oz), cut to fit into a saucepan (not aluminium or copper). Add 570mL (1 pint) of filtered rainwater and bring to the boil. Simmer for 30 minutes. Liquid is reduced to about half (285mL or approximately ½ pint). Cool, strain and bottle. Store in the refrigerator for up to 3 days.

MACERATION

Herbs that are likely to lose their therapeutic properties if heated can be steeped in oil, vinegar or alcohol. Pack a glass bottle with crushed, fresh herbs and cover with vegetable oil, cider vinegar or pure alcohol. Avoid leaves in oil as they tend to rot. Seal and leave for 2 weeks, shaking bottle daily. Strain and top up with fresh herbs. Repeat until the liquid smells strongly herbal. Strain, seal and bottle.

PULVERISATION

Grind, bruise or mash plant fibres and seeds in a mortar and pestle or electric blender. Pulverised herb can be used as a poultice by placing between gauze (Bremness, 1988).

Useful Herbs

If you are using herbs for medicinal purposes please consult with a naturopath or herbalist prior to commencement as some herbs may work against a pre-existing condition or an underlying ailment that you are unaware of, producing a much larger condition to then have to deal with. Be wise and see a trained herbalist. There are 1,000's of herbs on this planet that are useful and so much information available on each one far beyond what I have only touched on here. For more information, please refer to Useful Websites.

ALFALFA Medicago sativa

Rich in vitamins, alfalfa contains 8 essential amino acids, and 8 essential digestive enzymes that are known to promote chemical reactions enabling food to be assimilated accurately within the body. Alfalfa contains vitamins A, B, E, K, and D and is high in protein, contains phosphorous, iron, potassium, chlorine, sodium, silicon, magnesium and other trace elements. A hormone herb, alfalfa may stabilise calcium, eliminate retained water; treat recuperative cases of narcotic and alcohol addiction. Alfalfa, named by the Arabs centuries ago, means "Father of all Foods" because they claimed that it made their animals (such as horses) swift and strong. Alfalfa is said to possess no unfriendly components so may be given to children, adults, and nursing mothers. As a tea alfalfa is pleasant when combined with spearmint or peppermint.

CEDARWOOD Cedrus atlantica (Coniferae)

Cedarwood may be used as a fungicide on dandruff, skin disorders and ulcers, anti-seborrheic on oily hair, and for inducing deep relaxation.

CHAMOMILE Anthemis nobilis (Compositae)

Chamomile derives its name from the Greek kamai (on the ground) and melon (apple). Chamomile tea may relieve an upset stomach, cold, bronchitis, bladder troubles, dropsy, and jaundice; may regulate menstrual cycle, rheumatic pains, headache, and hysteria; may remedy a child's restlessness and fever; is a good wash for sore eyes, open sores and wounds; as a gargle for sore throats; sponged over the body acts as an insect repellent; tea rinse for blond hair; an additive for a calming bath; and the dried flowers add a delicate aroma among linen.

COMFREY Symphytum officinale

High in calcium, potassium, phosphorus, and other trace minerals, comfrey also contains protein and vitamins A, C and B12; is high in lysine, an amino acid usually lacking in a meat-free diet. Other vitamins found are B1, B2, niacin, pantothenic acid (B5), D, E, and choline. Comfrey contains the healing agent allantoin, known to promote granulation and formation of epithelial cells, thus increasing nature's speed of healing a wound, internal irritation, or broken bone. Seek naturopathic advice before taking internally. A decoction added to a bath also tones the skin.

DANDELION Taraxacum officinale

Dandelion increases liver, pancreas and spleen activity. With high vitamin and mineral content, it may be useful for treating kidney and liver disorders and loss of appetite. Young leaves can be used in salads, and larger leaves cooked as a vegetable. Ground dried and roasted roots make a coffee substitute.

EUCALYPTUS Eucalyptus globulus Myrtaceae)

The microbial properties of eucalyptol in an infusion is used as a safe antiseptic; for soothing inflamed mucous membranes; and relieving asthma and croup. A few drops of oil on a small cloth and inhaled may relieve a congested head. Be aware that too much inhalation can also create sores in the back of the nose.

GOLDEN SEAL Hydrastis canadensis

Golden Seal has a very positive effect on the mucous membranes and body tissues, being helpful with most external sores and inflammations. Golden Seal infusion used as a douche also soothes inflammations of the vagina and uterus. Golden Seal will help to alleviate sore gums when brushed with a tea infusion. A cooled infusion can be applied to an inflamed eye. After washing skin ailments with an infusion, sprinkle with powdered root. Persons with hypoglycaemia, hypertension or are pregnant must seek medical advice prior to using Golden Seal internally.

HOREHOUND Marrubrium vulgare

Horehound as a tea is used for cough and cold treatments.

KELP Fucus vesiculosus

Kelp treats the thyroid gland.

LAVENDER Lavandula officinalis (Labiatae)

Lavender is an antiseptic, and is calming on the nervous system. The dried flowers are used in perfumery and as aromatic sachets amongst clothing, also repelling insects.

LEMON Citrus limonom (Rutaceae)

Lemon may control the liquid processes of the lymphatic system and secretions; is a tonic on the nervous system; uplifting on anaemia, anxiety and depression.

LEMONGRASS Cymbogogon citratus (Graminae)

Astringent and tonic on open pores; deodoriser and disinfectant; stimulates digestion. As an essential oil Lemongrass can irritant the skin.

LIME Citrus limetta (Rutaceae)

Lime is refreshing as a drink in hot climates when mixed with chilled filtered, detoxified rainwater. Lime may control the liquid processes of the lymphatic system and secretions; is a tonic on the nervous system; uplifting on anaemia, anxiety and depression.

LIQUORICE Glycyrrhiza glabra

Liquorice (the herb itself, not the sugary sweet) treats the respiratory system; can be used as a laxative; and has anti-inflammatory qualities.

MELISSA Melissa officinalis (Labiatae)

This uplifting and soothing herb is also antiseptic and cythophylactic on acne, eczema and dermatitis; stimulates the metabolism and the vital centres; is calming and sedative on insomnia, migraine and nervous tension; appeasing on the astral body and stimulates the heart chakra.

MILK THISTLE Silybum marianum

Milk thistle is used to treat leg ulcers and hepatitis.

MYRRH Commiphora myrrha (Burseraceae)

Myrrh is cooling and drying on inflammations and infected wounds, regulates secretions. Myrrh stimulates the third eye and crown chakras.

NEROLI Citrus vulgaris (Rutaceae)

Neroli stimulates the heart chakra; is an anti-depressant and sedative on emotional shock and grief. Neroli is soothing on sensitive skin; hypotensor and sedative on palpitations.

PEPPERMINT Mentha piperita (Labiatae)

Peppermint is invigorating, cleanses and strengthens the entire internal body, including the nerves when taken as an infusion. Peppermint may be useful against flatulence, dizziness, seasickness, nausea, vomiting, chills, colic, fevers, diarrhoea, influenza and indigestion. As an enema, peppermint may be useful for colon troubles. Peppermint oil may be soothing on toothache and rheumatism.

SLIPPERY ELM Ulmus fulva

Slippery Elm is rich in mucilage and soothes inflamed surfaces, helps heal gastric ulcers and helps control diarrhoea.

SPEARMINT Mentha viridis (Labiatae)

Spearmint is a cleanser and decongestant on acne, decongestant on sinuses, and calming on the stomach.

TARRAGON French Artemisia dracunculus (Compositae)

Tarragon is an antispasmodic and digestive on digestive and intestinal spasms, dyspepsia and hiccup. Tarragon is used to flavour Bernaise sauce, chicken, fish, and salads.

TEA TREE Melaleaca alternifolia (Myrtaceae)

Tea Tree is a well-known general antiseptic and fungicide.

UVA URSI Bearberry Arctostaphylos uva-ursi

Bearberry may treat urinary disorders such as bladder and kidney infections, urinary incontinence and acute cystitis.

VANILLA Vanilla planifolia

Vanilla is a popular flavouring used widely in cookery and perfumery.

YLANG YLANG Cananga odorata genuine

Ylang Ylang has an exotic aroma that is calming and sedative.

THE AUTHOR

This journey into the world of therapeutic massage began at the age of fifteen however I was unaware of it until in my thirties. After painful and uncontrollable cramps engulfed my entire body, twisting arms and legs and torso too, Mum and Dad came to my rescue. They took one leg each, stretched them out until the cramps released, only to be followed by another and another, and another and another…

As the contractions began to ease, massage was used to ease the intense pain that remained in the muscles. Without massage I was unable to walk for two days. Massaging came as a natural instinct to them both. It takes two, the giver and the receiver to help remove pain from the body. The more there is of giving, the results are more healing if the receiver is willing to accept being healed. I am fortunate to have been blessed with parents who gave so much of themselves when I most needed them.

Between the ages of six and thirty, numerous tests, x-rays, injections of drugs and operations were performed, many drugs consumed, five weeks spent in a neuro-psychiatric hospital to 'dry out' from some of these prescribed drugs, a few more weeks in hospital under the care of psychiatrists, an exorcism and the stopping of my heart beat, I realised after all this that the best form of healing is therapeutic massage, coupled with positive heavenly spirit, inner calm (by regular meditation), rain water and down to earth goodness given by Mother Nature – the 'fruits' of the earth – food. Positive affirmations in meditation and song commenced in 1988. Since that time the need for pain killers ceased with less than one packet being taken to this very day. With twenty-seven years of living proof behind me, I certainly can vouch for the healing and balancing power of forgiveness, meditation and positive affirmations. Many years have been lived since then to prove this works best for dissolving inner angers, resentments and grievances which cause nearly every pain and illness that are derived from destructive, negative words and actions. I feel that I was chosen to come through each of these experiences and arrive on the good side of life again to share some of the numerous gentle healing techniques with others.

We can either choose to think thoughts that create a mental atmosphere that contributes to illness or we can all choose to think thoughts that create a healthy atmosphere. It feels so good to have discovered this more healthy way of living – balancing the body, mind and spirit, being as one, being grateful for my body, loving life knowing that all the changes that lie before me in life are now positive ones.

October 14th, 1987 saw the commencement of the first of five therapeutic massage centres. Marketing the business was very intense due to the negative connotations around the word 'massage'. The many calls, sniggers and comments that came were characterised by the union of male and female. Best of all to emerge from my continual driving persistence that therapeutic massage is for healing was the influx of people with real physical issues. Within a short space in time my first staff member was employed. Recommendations for treatments came from doctors, physiotherapists, chiropractors, social workers, ministers and naturopaths. The necessity of teaching began in 1988 due to a demand for the higher Holistic approach to wellness and my college of therapeutic massage opened in January, 1990. The Australian Massage therapy video, cassette and training manual were produced for the college also in 1990.

After seeing the Health Minister for Queensland with regards to recognition of therapeutic massage I was told to 'get the ball rolling' by collecting many signatures from people requesting this. After commencing petitions in 1988, it was during the following year I presented many pages of signatures to health funds requesting that therapeutic massage be recognised within Australia's health system.

When Queensland Association of Massage Therapists (QAMT) affiliated with Australian Association of Massage Therapists (AAMT) my trained practitioners were directed to join this Australia wide association. AAMT displayed a progressive nature leading qualified massage therapists to be eligible, like others in the medical profession who have substantial studies backing and supporting them, to health benefit rebates for the distinguished service they performed. I have long believed that a professional therapeutic back massage once a month combined with daily, positive, health-creating affirmations are an inspiration to the energetic inputs within our great country, freeing so many from fearful, negative thought patterns.

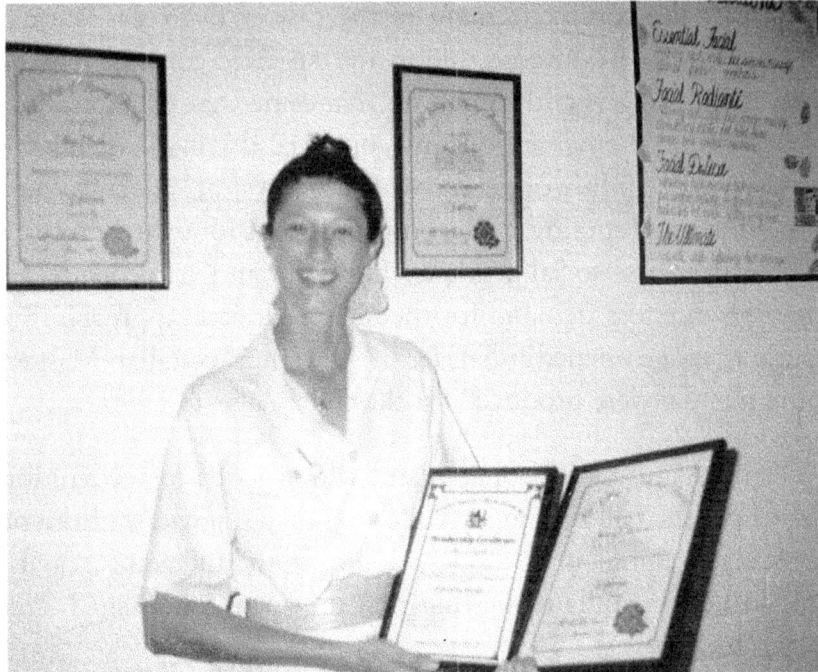

Diploma, Certificates and
Therapist Registration 1987

Today Certificate IV qualified massage practitioners are recognised as professional in our health industry. I feel honoured to have played a small part in this major event. The process engaged many people Australia wide who strongly believed in the benefits of remedial massage. Years have now passed and therapeutic massage performed by professionally qualified practitioners is readily accepted as a natural part of one's well-being by numerous health funds Australia wide.

With or without rebates, increasing numbers of the general public who are seeking massage therapy show that people do prefer to make healthier choices, have more respect for themselves, want to be pain free naturally and still be totally in sync with life. They are doing their best at creating perfect health and are looking forward to a healthy old age because they are taking care of their bodies now. By going within they connect with that part of themselves that knows how to heal. This is where miracles commence, going within and loving the self.

I became a member of the Queensland Association of Massage Therapists Incorporated (QAMT) in 1987 after receiving the first in a series of qualifications from the Queensland College of Massage Therapy, and then following QAMT affiliation with all States in Australia, the Australian Association of Massage Therapists (AAMT) from 2003.

On the 8th February, 1999 I was awarded an official Certificate of Accreditation for Course in Natural Health which became a nationally recognised training product from 1999 to 2004. This Course complied with the requirements of the Australian Recognition Framework and the Vocational Education, Training and Employment Commission (VETEC), and since then has ceased due to my pursuit of providing healthier beverages into stores.

The Australian Massage method continues to be accepted today in health centres, day spas and beauty salons in Australia, England, Europe, Asia and United States of America. I hope you have enjoyed this method too. When searching for a qualified practitioner, simply begin by asking friends who they are happy with or refer to an accredited Association in your country.

REFERENCES

Ahimsa (Online), Available: www.ahimsaoils.com.au

Bijlsma, Nicole 2010, "Certificate IV in Building Biology," Australian College of Environmental Studies, Suite 2 / 25-29 Prospect St, Box Hill, VIC, 3128, (Online), Available: www.buildingbiology.com or www.aces.edu.au

Birnbaum, Linda S. and Staskal, Daniele F. 2004, 'Brominated flame retardants: cause for concern?' Environmental Health Perspectives, vol. 112, no. 1, pp. 9-17 (Online), Available: www.ncbi.nlm.nih.gov/.../v.112(1); Jan 2004

Bremness, Lesley 1988, The Complete Book of Herbs, pg 213 "Basic Herbal Preparations," Book, ISBN 0 86438 066 6, © Dorling Kindersley Limited, 9 Henrietta Street, London WC2E 8PS, Reprinted 1991, 1992. (Online), Available: at time of writing, www.amazon.com/

California Department of Public Health, 2011, Indoor Air Quality Program, A Brief Guide to Mold, Moisture, and Your Home, "Mold Basics,"(Online), Available: http://www.epa.gov/mold/moldbasics.html

"Mold Cleanup Guidelines," (Online), Available: http://www.epa.gov/mold/cleanupguidelines.html

"About Mold and Dampness," (Online), Available: http://www.cal-iaq.org/mold/about-mold

Calvert, Robert Noah 1987, Pages from History, "Notations of the General Principles of Gymnastics by Pehr Henrik Ling," Lars Agren and Patricia Benjamin, trans.

Journal of the American Massage Therapy Association, (Online), Available: http://www.massagemag.com/Magazine/2002/issue100/history100.php

Dust Mite Information Centre, 2004, (Online), Available: http://www..com/findmites.htm

dust-mite.net, 2012 (Online), Available: http://www.dust-mite.net/dust-mite-control/

Grant, Lucinda 1997, "Electrical Sensitivity as an Emerging Illness," (Online), Available: http://www.tldp.com/issue/179/emf179.htm

Hay, Louise L. 1984, You Can heal Your Life, "Deep at the centre of my being there is an infinite well of love," (Online), Available: www.hayhouse.com.au

Lorber, M 2007, 'Exposure of Americans to polybrominated diphenyl ethers,' Journal of Exposure Science and Environmental Epidemiology, vol. 18 (Online), Available: www.mendeley.com/.../exposure-americans-polybromin...-United States

Minnesota Dept. of Health, 2011 Formaldehyde in Your Home, "What is Formaldehyde," Where is it found?" "What can be done to reduce the formaldehyde level?" (Online), Available: http://www.health.state.mm.us/divs/eh/indoorair/voc/formaldehyde.htm

Minnesota Department of Health, June 2012, Mold and Moisture in Homes, "What are the health concerns?" "Are the risks greater for some people?" "Are some molds more hazardous than others?" "Home Investigation," "Should I test for mold?" Mold Clean-up and Removal," (Online), Available: http://www.health.state.mn.us/divs/eh/indoorair/mold/index/htm;

NCRP Scientific Committee, 1995, 89-3: "Draft Report on Extremely Low Frequency Electric and Magnetic Fields, July/August 1995, p.12-15. (Online), Available: http://www.equilibrauk.com/emfsbio.shtml

Powerwatch Appliances Factsheet 2012, (Online), Available: www.powerwatch.org.uk/elf/appliances.asp

Russell, 2001, Fragrance Sensitivity, 2001 (Online), Available: allnaturalbeauty.us/chemicalsensitivities

Chemical Sensitivities and Perfume, Chemicals and Pesticides, (Online), Available: allnaturalbeauty.us/chemicalsensitivities, then http://jrussellshealth.org

Rutherford, Teresa, "Compost Happens", Online, trutherford@ozemail.com.au

"Scientific Facts About ElectromagneticRadiation" (Online), Available: www.rainforestinfo.org.au/good_wood/emr_fact.htm

Shekut, Sue 2009, (Online), Available: workingwellresources.com/.../nasas-top-ten-plants-to-remove-formal...

U.S. House of Representatives, 1986, "Neurotoxins: At Home and the Workplace," Report by the Committee on Science & Technology, Sept. 16, 1986, (Report 99-827) (Online), Available: www.herc.org/news/perfume/scents.htm

Yvonne, 2010 Plants Absorb Indoor Pollution Online, www.earthwitchery.com/pollution.html

Ziem, Grace M.D. 2001, Chemical Awareness, "Why Scents Don't Make Sense," (Online), Available: http://www.ecoviva.com/html/synthetic-fragrances.html

USEFUL WEBSITES

Allergy and Environmental Sensitivity Support and Research Association, AESSRA, 2008 Chemical sensitivity and MCS, (Online), Available: www.aessra.org/chemical-sensitivity-and-mcs.php

Anatomy and Charts, (Online), Available: www.medshop.com.au

Antol, Marie Nadine 1996, Book, Healing Teas, "A Practical Guide to the Medicinal Teas of the World – From Chamomile to Garlic, From Essiac to Kombucha," "How to Prepare and Use Teas to Maximize Your Health," (Online), Available: at time of writing, www.amazon.com/

Aromatherapy Products, (Online), Available: www.perfect potion.com.au

Battaglia, Salvatore 1995, The Complete Guide to Aromatherapy (Online), Available: www.perfectpotion.com.au

Bijlsma, Nicole 2010, Book, Healthy Home Healthy Family, "Chemicals, Chemicals Everywhere!" Pg 241- 2 Available: www.aces.edu.au

Bridges Betty, n.d. Practical Asthma Reviews, Fragrances and Chemical Sensitivities, (Online), Available: www.ameliaww.com/fpin/fpin.htm

Clotfelter, Susan n.d., Book, The Herb Tea Book, "Blending, Brewing and Savoring Teas for

Every Meal and Occasion," (Online), Available: at time of writing, www.amazon.com/

Dewey David Lawrence, 1999, Food For Thought, Colognes – Perfumes – Pesticides, Are They Slowly Killing You? (Online), Available: www.dldewey.com/perfume.htm

Dunne, Lavon J. 1990, Book, Nutrition Almanac Third Edition, Nutrition Search, Inc. Kirschmann, John D. Director, (Online), Available: at time of writing, www.amazon.com/

Grieve, Mrs M. 1994, A Modern Herbal (Online), Available at time of writing at www.abebooks.co.uk/book-search/...modern-herbal/...mrs.m.grieve/...

Gruenberg, Louise 1999, Book, Herbal Home Hints, Rodale's Essential Herbal Handbooks, "Hundreds of Tips and Formulas for Cleaning just about Anything," (Online), Available: at time of writing, www.amazon.com/

Health Risks of Perfume, April 2002, (Online), Available: www.ourlittleplace.com

Hopman, Ellen Evert 1995, Book, A Druid's Herbal for the Sacred Earth Year, (Online), Available at time of writing, www.amazon.com/

Lavabre, Marcel F. 1990, Aromatherapy Workbook ISBN 0 89281 346 6 Healing Arts Press, One Park Street, Rochester, Vermont 05767 www.amazon.com/ may have a copy available

Marcin, Marietta Marshall 1999, Herbal Tea Gardens, "22 Plans for your Enjoyment and Well-Being," (Online), Available: at time of writing, www.amazon.com/

Parker, James W. 1975, Parker Chiropractic Research Foundation, Parker University, Parker Chiropractic Wellness Clinics, (Online), Available, www.parker.edu/chiropractic.aspx?ia=401

Tortora, Grabowski: Principles of Anatomy and Physiology (Online), Available: www.wiley.com/legacy/college/bio/tortora366927/.../student/ and www.wiley.com/college/tortora

Virtue, Doreen Ph.D., Spiritual doctor of psychology (Online), Available: www.AngelTherapy.com

For more life improvements, such as Creating Wellness, Good Health, Relationships, Work Success and Prosperity please visit www.paradisewaters1.com

RECOMMENDATIONS

Rainwater

RAINFOREST DEW™, Mother Nature's Premium Rainwater. It's made in Heaven and North Queensland.

Oxygenated, ultra-finely filtered, with a molecular structure that allows full absorption of oxygen, therefore hydration can contribute to an environment primarily desirable for physical wellbeing, creating an inner glow.

10 Litres - with tap for easy access - in-house, groups, on-sites, bench tops

5 Litres - for a crowd, on the road, in the boat, caravan…

1.5L - table & travel

600mL - goes everywhere –companion

600mL - with SPORT cap - for hand free opening

350mL - with SPORT cap

350mL - thirst quencher

Available:

Paradise Waters Pty Ltd

www.rainforestdewonline.com

Music for All Occasions

Available:

Lifestyle Music

 "Nature, Meditation, Health & Wellbeing, Classical, Spa"

www.lifestylemusic.com.au

Natural Cleaning Aids

Available:

Abode

www.buildingbiology.com.au

Accommodation

Available:

Romantic Retreats

www.romanticretreats.com.au

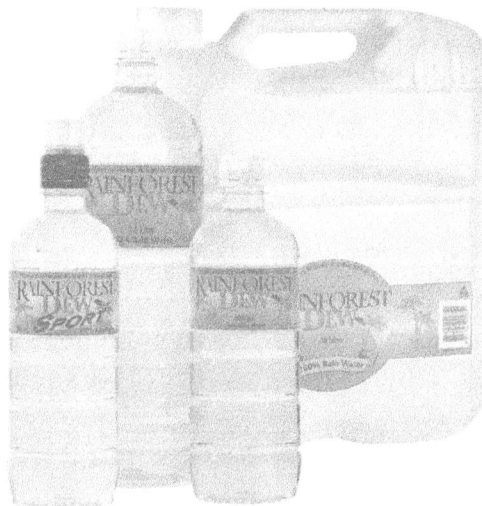

THE BEST FROM THE LIBRARY OF NANCY F. HEGARTY/NEWITT

CDs

DAILY RELAXATION MEDITATION

For re-energising, re-balancing and gentle healing this is a must if you are in the healing profession, feel overworked or stuck in life. Rise from this session feeling the amazing benefits. This is not your average every day relaxation meditation.

PAIN MANAGEMENT & PREPARATION FOR HEALING

This meditation will create a healthy atmosphere for both within you and around you. If you are willing to accept new thoughts healing can happen.

MEDITATION FOR MUSTERING INTENSIVE ENERGY

Feel the power as you draw upon the 12th Chakra Universal Cosmic Energy while in a higher state of consciousness and expand beyond any limitations in your life.

AN INTRODUCTION TO A HEALTHY LIFE

The Most Loving 286 Life Affirmations, the Gift to Creating Miracles is easy listening at home and play, going to and from work. Experience the freedom as you create an even more enjoyable life.

EBooks

THE AUSTRALIAN MASSAGE... Feeling the Healing
Practical movements for the beginner
Enhancing skills for the experienced practitioner
Professional instructions with many intricate, close-up photographs
Originally produced for students at Australian colleges

SIMPLE FOODS TO HEAL YOUR BODY

Recommended for permanent healing guidance

Shows delicious healing foods for ailments A to Z

Keep this instant guide with you when shopping for food if you have any ailment; look up the ailment that is listed from A to Z, then choose the foods that you like to enhance the healing process and enjoy eating your way to better health; includes a hint of Metaphysics and an introduction to Modern Feng Shui

THE AUSTRALIAN ADVANCED AND METAPHYSICAL MASSAGE

includes Proprioceptive Neuromuscular Facilitation Stretches (PNFs) to the Neck and Spine, Sciatic Release, Freeing the Shoulders, Releasing Knotted Muscles, Palm Release, Chopping and Pummelling Major Muscles, Shoulder, Elbow and Wrist Stretches, Hip, Knee and Ankle Stretches, Pre-Sports and Post Sports Massage, Pregnant Lady Massage Techniques, Hot Herbal Towel Applications, Metaphysics and the Body, Invigorating Affirmations for Re-Aligning Vertebrae and Spiritual Advancement. This expands in-depth appreciation for the basically trained beginner, and broadens the professional practitioner's experiences; includes an introduction to Kinesiology, Lymphatic Massage and Reflexology

BOOKs

THE AUSTRALIAN MASSAGE ... Feeling the Healing

Practical movements for the beginner

Enhancing skills for the experienced practitioner

Professional instructions with many intricate, close-up photographs

Originally produced for students at Australian colleges

SIMPLE FOODS TO HEAL YOUR BODY

Recommended for permanent healing guidance

Shows delicious healing foods for ailments A to Z

Keep this instant guide with you when shopping for food if you have any ailment; look up the ailment that is listed from A to Z, then choose the foods that you like to enhance the healing process and enjoy eating your way to better health; includes a hint of Metaphysics and an introduction to Modern Feng Shui

THE AUSTRALIAN ADVANCED AND METAPHYSICAL MASSAGE

includes Proprioceptive Neuromuscular Facilitation Stretches (PNFs) to the Neck and Spine, Sciatic Release, Freeing the Shoulders, Releasing Knotted Muscles, Palm Release, Chopping and Pummelling Major Muscles, Shoulder, Elbow and Wrist Stretches, Hip, Knee and Ankle Stretches, Pre-Sports and Post Sports Massage, Pregnant Lady Massage Techniques, Hot Herbal Towel Applications, Metaphysics and the Body, Invigorating Affirmations for Re-Aligning Vertebrae and Spiritual Advancement. This expands in-depth appreciation for the basically trained beginner, and broadens the professional practitioner's experiences; includes an introduction to Kinesiology, Lymphatic Massage and Reflexology

DVD

THE AUSTRALIAN MASSAGE THERAPY

Professional instructions with detailed practical movements for the beginner, and enhancing skills for the qualified practitioner

Pain Management & Preparation for Healing

PAIN MANAGEMENT & PREPARATION FOR HEALING

THIS MEDITATION WILL CREATE A HEALTHY ATMOSPHERE BOTH WITHIN YOU & AROUND YOU

Healing can happen!

Being pain free and totally synchronized with life is your Divine Right now. Listening and following this meditation has the power to prepare your body for healing and can create miracles in your life. *Pain Management & Preparation for Healing* is easy to follow enabling you to go within, connect with that part of you that knows how to heal and where you know pure love. Knowing each body cell has Divine intelligence, you listen to what it tells you and know that its advice is valid. You are always safe, protected and guided as you feel how your body wants to be healed.

Daily Relaxation Meditation

DAILY RELAXATION MEDITATION

FOR RE-ENERGISING RE-BALANCING and GENTLE HEALING

RE-ENERGISING

RE-BALANCING AND GENTLY HEALING

WITH

DAILY RELAXATION MEDITATION

You can rise from this session feeling its amazing benefits. This is not your average every day relaxation meditation. It really does provide a special technique and you don't have to do a thing. Just breathe and relax on a bed or comfortable mat and listen. Every experience is a success.

Meditation for Mustering Intensive Energy

MEDITATION FOR MUSTERING INTENSIVE ENERGY

A Higher State of Consciousness

FEELING THE POWER

FROM HIGH ABOVE

Drawing Upon the 12th Chakra Universal Cosmic Energy to Expand Beyond Any Limitations in Life

An Introduction to a Healthy Life

AN INTRODUCTION TO A HEALTHY LIFE

Easy Listening
At Home and Play, Going to and from Work and Sport

THE MOST LOVING 286 LIFE AFFIRMATIONS

THE GIFT TO CREATING MIRACLES

The key to discovering where good feelings emerge and the gift to creating miracles in your life is available in AN INTRODUCTION TO A HEALTHY LIFE. By listening regularly to AN INTRODUCTION TO A HEALTHY LIFE you'll be amazed and overjoyed to see how people, places, things and situations change. We anchor poor relationships, problems, illness and poverty more in place by talking about any of them. Now you can feel good about yourself. If any of your current beliefs consist of; I never have sufficient money, I'm sick, I'm fat, I'm ugly, I'm stuck in a miserable job or I'm just not good enough, then you may continue being stuck in that experience. Being under the laws of our own consciousness, our own thoughts, we attract specific experiences to us as a result of the way we think. Changing our thinking process also changes everything else in our lives. If we continue along our current pathway in life then it is because we believe what another tells us as true and are happy with their beliefs. AN INTRODUCTION TO A HEALTHY LIFE presents as the gift to creating miracles in your life. LIVE IN THE NOW. Now is the time to experience the freedom of creating a more enjoyable life. Begin making miracles. AN INTRODUCTION TO A HEALTHY LIFE gives all the necessary life affirmations that can guide you to better ways in life. Our bodies know how to heal when they are working in a happy, healthy mental atmosphere. Listening to AN INTRODUCTION TO A HEALTHY LIFE releases old negative patterns that will no longer limit you. Go for life!

Available: *www.paradisewaters1.com*

www.ingramcontent.com/pod-product-compliance
Lightning Source LLC
Chambersburg PA
CBHW080250030426
42334CB00023BA/2769